Andrew Malekoff, MSW
Robert Salmon, DSW
Dominique Moyse Steinberg, DSW
Editors

Making Joyful Noise: The Art, Science, and Soul of Group Work

Making Joyful Noise: The Art, Science, and Soul of Group Work has been co-published simultaneously as *Social Work with Groups*, Volume 29, Numbers 2/3 2006.

Pre-publication
REVIEWS,
COMMENTARIES,
EVALUATIONS . . .

"AN AMAZING COLLECTION. . . . A POWERFUL INTEGRATION OF THEORY AND PRACTICE!. . . . Several chapters have particular importance today. Steinberg's description of the four ingredients of good group work is fantastic. Goodman's chapter on the organization context and influence on group work practice should be required reading for all group workers. Malekoff's chapter on a poetry club for kids builds beautifully on Goodman's chapter as it illustrates the importance of working within the environmental and organisational context. It also demonstrates the power of the purposeful use of activity. Vicki Hallas' chapter describing her experience as a social work student, should be required for every student. This moving account highlights student difficulties in planning and working with groups when the agency and field instructor don't have group work skills. With the decline of group work education, her struggle will be familiar to many a group work student."

Timothy B. Kelly, PhD, MSW
Head of Social Work Division
Glasgow Caledonian University

More pre-publication
REVIEWS, COMMENTARIES, EVALUATIONS . . .

"A reader will learn about group work theory, skills, and practice and also about its under-utilized power as a human development and therapeutic medium able to counter feelings of alienation and loneliness and provide places for people to learn, practice, and experience connection and accomplishment with other people. Among the MANY EXCITING AND CREATIVE USES OF GROUPS included are: a poetry group for emotionally disturbed youngsters; the use of boxing with high-risk and offender youth to reduce violence; a self defense group for women; a caregiver support group for the elderly; and bereavement support for spouses whose partners were lost to cancer. Being reminded alone of the value of mutual aid and democratic values in a time of "individualism" run rampant is worth the price of the book. Useful across human services disciplines, this book HAS MUCH TO OFFER PRACTITIONERS, ADMINISTRATORS, TEACHERS, STAFF TRAINERS, AND FOR CURRICULUM DEVELOPMENT. Roselle Kurland would be pleased and we are indebted to the authors who remind us again of the power of groups, their effectiveness, and their efficiency. After all, life is with people!"

Ralph L. Dolgoff, MA, MSW, DSW
Professor
School of Social Work
University of Maryland

"This book is testimony to the fact that groupwork has no borders and that its power is a common denominator wherever in the world it is practised. From camp to poetry club, from boxing ring to women's self defence class, the 'joyfulness' in the book's title is amply illustrated. The book introduces us to engaging and honest accounts of groupwork from a broad range of contributors–academics, educators, practitioners and students. And, in this risk averse climate, we are encouraged to be bold in our groupwork practice. . . . *Making Joyful Noise* is TESTIMONY TO THE RESILIENCE OF GROUPWORK. IT CAN THRIVE."

Mark Doel, PhD, MA (Oxon), CQSW
Professor
Research Professor of Social Work
Centre for Health and Social Care Research
Sheffield Hallam University
England
Co-Editor, Groupwork Journal

Making Joyful Noise:
The Art, Science,
and Soul of Group Work

Making Joyful Noise: The Art, Science, and Soul of Group Work has been co-published simultaneously as *Social Work with Groups*, Volume 29, Numbers 2/3 2006.

Monographs from *Social Work with Groups*™

For additional information on these and other Haworth Press titles, including descriptions, tables of contents, reviews, and prices, use the QuickSearch catalog at http://www.HaworthPress.com.

1. *Co-Leadership in Social Work with Groups,* edited by Catherine P. Papell, DSW, and Beulah Rothman, DSW (Vol. 3, No. 4, 1981). *Explores the co-leadership phenomenon in the experience of social work students studying groupwork.*

2. *Social Groupwork and Alcoholism,* edited by Marjorie Altman and Ruth Crocker (Vol. 5, No. 1, 1982). *"Useful information about a number of different kinds of groups in the treatment of alcoholism." (International Journal of Group Psychotherapy)*

3. *Groupwork with the Frail Elderly,* edited by Shura Saul, EdD, CSW (Vol. 5, No. 2, 1982). *"A rich mixture of different types of groups for frail elderly, and for those working with the frail elderly. . . . A valuable aid to social workers, nurses, or any professional working with such groups of individuals." (Journal of Gerontological Nursing)*

4. *The Use of Group Services in Permanency Planning for Children,* edited by Sylvia K. Morris, MSW (Vol. 5, No. 4, 1982). *This important sourcebook examines the use of social group work in establishing out-of-home children in permanent homes in an age of federal cutbacks.*

5. *Activities and Action in Groupwork,* edited by Ruth Middleman, EdD, MSW (Vol. 6, No. 1, 1983). *A very helpful resource on the use of activities in social groupwork with a variety of populations.*

6. *Groupwork with Women/Groupwork with Men: An Overview of Gender Issues in Social Groupwork Practice,* edited by Beth Glover Reed, PhD, and Charles D. Garvin, PhD (Vol. 6, No. 3/4, 1983). *"A variety of approaches to gender-sensitive groupwork, as well as applications of specific techniques in groups." (Social Work Reporter)*

7. *Ethnicity in Social Group Work Practice,* edited by Larry E. Davis (Vol. 7, No. 3, 1984). *"Excellent resource. . . . Will serve as a good supplemental text in a generic social group work course or as a main text in a specialized course." (Howard J. Doueck, Social Work Department, State University of New York at Buffalo)*

8. *Groupwork with Children and Adolescents,* edited by Ralph L. Kolodny, MA, MSSS, and James A. Garland, ACSW (Vol. 7, No. 4, 1984). *"Integrates time-tested models and procedures with emerging theories and models in a field where a paucity of material exists. . . . Should be of considerable interest to educators as well as social workers." (Voice of Youth Advocates)*

9. *Time as a Factor in Groupwork: Time-Limited Group Experiences,* edited by Albert S. Alissi, DSW, and Max Casper (Vol. 8, No. 2, 1985). *This informative book provides the helping professional with valuable information on the benefits and drawbacks of time-limited social groupwork.*

10. *The Legacy of William Schwartz: Group Practice as Shared Interaction,* edited by Alex Gitterman, EdD, MSW, and Lawrence Schulman (Vol. 8, No. 4, 1986). *This fine volume celebrates William Schwartz's lasting contribution to teaching and scholarship and conveys the power of his ideas and their relevance to contemporary practice.*

11. *Innovations in Social Group Work: Feedback from Practice to Theory,* edited by Marvin Parnes, MSW (Supplement #1, 1986). *This classic volume illustrates just how vigorous and inventive social groupwork can be.*

12. *Research in Social Group Work,* edited by Sheldon D. Rose, PhD, and Ronald A. Feldman (Vol. 9, No. 3, 1986). *Reflects not only on the important advances and strengths in group work research but also some of the deficiencies and gaps that characterize contemporary research in the field.*

13. *Collectivity in Social Group Work: Concept and Practice,* edited by Norma C. Lang, PhD, and Joanne Sulman, MSW (Vol. 9, No. 4, 1986). *A concise and comprehensive examination of the theory of collectivity in social group work.*

14. *Working Effectively with Administrative Groups,* edited by Ronald W. Toseland, PhD, and Paul H. Ephross, PhD (Vol. 10, No. 2, 1987). *Exciting suggestions for making administrative groups more effective.*

15. *Social Group Work: Competence and Values in Practice,* edited by Joseph Lassner, PhD, MSW, Kathleen Powell, MSW, and Elaine Finnegan, MSW (Supplement #2, 1987). *Detailed information on group work theory, group structure, gender and race issues in group work, group work in health care settings, and the use of groups for coping with family issues that will be invaluable for all professionals in their daily practice.*

16. *Violence: Prevention and Treatment in Groups,* edited by George S. Getzel, DSW (Vol. 11, No. 3, 1988). *"A useful supplement for a library serving a social work, mental health, or family therapy curriculum." (Academic Library Book Review)*

17. *Group Work with the Poor and Oppressed,* edited by Judith A. B. Lee, DSW (Vol. 11, No. 4, 1988). *"A rich source of reference material for those looking for historical, theoretical, and practical references." (Australian Social Work)*

18. *Roots and New Frontiers in Social Group Work,* by Marcus Leiderman, MSW, Martin L. Birnbaum, PhD, and Barbara Dazzo, PhD (Supplement #3, 1989). *"The vitality of contemporary social group work is reflected in this book. . . . A worthwhile contribution to the literature." (Social Work)*

19. *Social Work with Multi-Family Groups,* edited by D. Rosemary Cassano, PhD, MSW (Vol. 12, No. 1, 1989). *Better understand the interrelatedness of the primary family group and the formed therapeutic group with this book.*

20. *Groups in Health Care Settings,* edited by Janice H. Schopler, PhD, and Maeda J. Galinsky, PhD (Vol. 12, No. 4, 1989). *"This timely collection offers a broad ranging view of what's happening through groups in hospitals and community agencies." (Ruth R. Middleman, EdD, ACSW, Professor, Kent School of Social Work, University of Louisville)*

21. *Group Work with the Emotionally Disabled,* edited by Baruch Levine, PhD (Vol. 13, No. 1, 1990). *"Provides an excellent overview of group work within a variety of settings and with a variety of populations." (Adult Residential Care Journal)*

22. *Ethnicity and Biculturalism: Emerging Perspectives of Social Group Work,* edited by Kenneth L. Chau, PhD (Vol. 13, No. 4, 1991). *"Offers a tremendous help in focusing on the issues and addresses them in a straightforward manner. It is highly recommended for those in 'helping' professions." (Multiculture Publishers Exchange Newsletter)*

23. *Groupwork with Suburbia's Children: Difference, Acceptance, and Belonging,* edited by Andrew Malekoff, MSW (Vol. 14, No. 1, 1991). *"Provide[s] a careful, professional look into the multiple problems of the children and youth outside of the inner city and minority areas in which we traditionally expect to find such problems." (Social Work with Groups Newsletter)*

24. *Theory and Practice in Social Group Work: Creative Connections,* edited by Marie Weil, DSW, Kenneth L. Chau, PhD, and Dannia Southerland, MSW (Supplement #4, 1991). *Here is an important look at creative ways to successfully blend theoretical knowledge with skillful intervention in social group work.* Theory and Practice in Social Group Work *represents leading works in conceptual development that creatively connect practice with theory and also reflect the current diversity of interventions in group work practice.*

25. *Social Action in Group Work,* edited by Abe Vinik and Morris Levin (Vol. 14, No. 3/4, 1992). *"Focuses on getting rid of the causes of problems through group action. . . . Numerous examples are provided for students, educators, researchers, and practitioners." (Social Work with Groups Newsletter)*

26. *Group Work Reaching Out: People, Places, and Power,* edited by James A. Garland, AB, MSSS (Vol. 15, No. 2/3, 1992). *"Experienced leaders in practice and teaching of social work*

with groups address the problems and potential of a wide variety of vulnerable, alienated, underserved, and politically disenfranchised populations. . . . A must." (Social Work with Groups Newsletter)

27. **Social Work with Groups: Expanding Horizons,** edited by Stanley Wenocur, PhD, Thomas Vassil, PhD, Paul Ephross, PhD, and Raju Varghese, EdD, MPH (Vol. 16, No. 1/2, 1993). *"Fascinating and interesting. The chapters are excellent, spanning theory and direct practice with groups. . . . Helpful to practitioners and educators. I recommend it highly to both." (Joan K. Parry, DSW, LCSW, Professor, College of Social Work, San Jose State University)*

28. **Support Groups: Current Perspectives on Theory and Practice,** edited by Maeda J. Galinsky, PhD, and Janice H. Schopler, PhD (Vol. 18, No. 1, 1996). *"Provides a framework for understanding and examining supportive group interventions. Provides descriptions of different kinds of support groups and alerts practitioners and educators to issues of planning, implementing, and evaluating such services." (The Brown University Child and Adolescent Behavior Newsletter)*

29. **Voices from the Field: Group Work Responds,** edited by Albert S. Alissi, DSW, and Catherine G. Corto Mergins, MSW (1997). *"Group workers, agencies, and undergraduate and graduate social work programs will want to act quickly to add this important collection to their libraries. . . .The contributors make significant new knowledge, values, and skills available for group workers everywhere." (Social Work with Groups Newsletter)*

30. **Rebuilding Communities: Challenges for Group Work,** edited by Harvey Bertcher, DSW, Linda Farris Kurtz, DPA, and Alice Lamont, PhD (1999). *"Demonstrates the many ways in which group work intervention techniques can be employed to improve communities, groups, families, and individuals. The strength of this volume for social workers is rooted in the excellent chapters that describe the versatility of group work by illuminating the wide range of possible clients that can be assisted through the systematic application of its intervention techniques." (Sustainable Communities Review)*

31. **Stories Celebrating Group Work: It's Not Always Easy to Sit on Your Mouth,** edited by Roselle Kurland, PhD, and Andrew Malekoff, ACSW (Vol. 25, No. 1/2, 2002). *"A rare glimpse at some of the crucial moments that have inspired, influenced, and created real groupworkers." (Lainey Collins, CSW, Camp Director, The Fresh Air Fund)*

32. **A Quarter Century of Classics (1978-2004): Capturing the Theory, Practice, and Spirit of Social Work with Groups,** edited by Andrew Malekoff, MSW, and Roselle Kurland, PhD (Vol. 28, No. 3/4, 2006). *"Students and instructors will value this book tremendously. Finally, in one book are several seminal papers on group work theory and practice that have appeared in Social Work wih Groups. The editors made wise and thoughtful choices; each chapter contributes strongly to the whole. Students of group work, faculty members, and social work scholars will not go wrong by purchasing this text and referring to it in their work. THIS IS A WONDERFUL TEXT!" (Meredith Hanson, DSW, Director, PhD in Social Work Program, Fordham University Graduate School of Social Service)*

33. **Making Joyful Noise: The Art, Science, and Soul of Group Work,** edited by Andrew Malekoff, MSW, Robert Salmon, DSW, and Dominique Moyse Steinberg, DSW (Vol. 29, No. 2/3, 2006). *A special collection on the power and joy of group work.*

Making Joyful Noise: The Art, Science, and Soul of Group Work

Andrew Malekoff, MSW
Robert Salmon, DSW
Dominique Moyse Steinberg, DSW
Editors

With Foreword by Helen Northen

Making Joyful Noise: The Art, Science, and Soul of Group Work has been co-published simultaneously as *Social Work with Groups*, Volume 29, Numbers 2/3 2006.

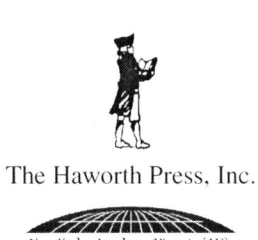

The Haworth Press, Inc.

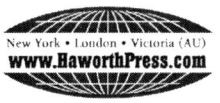

New York • London • Victoria (AU)
www.HaworthPress.com

Published by

The Haworth Press, Inc., 10 Alice Street, Binghamton, NY 13904-1580 USA

Making Joyful Noise: The Art, Science, and Soul of Group Work has been co-published simultaneously as *Social Work with Groups*, Volume 29, Numbers 2/3 2006.

The development, preparation, and publication of this work has been undertaken with great care. However, the publisher, employees, editors, and agents of The Haworth Press and all imprints of The Haworth Press, Inc., including The Haworth Medical Press® and The Pharmaceutical Products Press®, are not responsible for any errors contained herein or for consequences that may ensue from use of materials or information contained in this work. With regard to case studies, identities and circumstances of individuals discussed herein have been changed to protect confidentiality. Any resemblance to actual persons, living or dead, is entirely coincidental.

The Haworth Press is committed to the dissemination of ideas and information according to the highest standards of intellectual freedom and the free exchange of ideas. Statements made and opinions expressed in this publication do not necessarily reflect the views of the Publisher, Directors, management, or staff of The Haworth Press, Inc., or an endorsement by them.

Cover design by Jennifer Gaska.

Library of Congress Cataloging-in-Publication Data

Making joyful noise: the art, science, and soul of group work / Andrew Malekoff, Robert Salmon, Dominique Moyse Steinberg, editors.
     p. cm.
     "... co-published simultaneously as Social work with groups, volume 29, numbers 2/3, 2006."
     Includes bibliographical references.
     ISBN-13: 978-0-7890-3237-9 (hard cover : alk. paper)
     ISBN-10: 0-7890-3237-6 (hard cover : alk. paper)
     ISBN-13: 978-0-7890-3238-6 (soft cover : alk. paper)
     ISBN-10: 0-7890-3238-4 (soft cover : alk. paper)
     1. Social group work. I. Malekoff, Andrew II. Salmon, Robert. III. Steinberg, Dominique Moyse. IV. Social work with groups (Haworth Press)

HV45.M32 2006
361.4–dc22
                                               2006015774

Indexing, Abstracting & Website/Internet Coverage

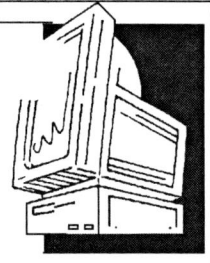

This section provides you with a list of major indexing & abstracting services and other tools for bibliographic access. That is to say, each service began covering this periodical during the year noted in the right column. Most Websites which are listed below have indicated that they will either post, disseminate, compile, archive, cite or alert their own Website users with research-based content from this work. (This list is as current as the copyright date of this publication.)

(continued)

(continued)

(continued)

Special Bibliographic Notes related to special journal issues (separates) and indexing/abstracting:

- indexing/abstracting services in this list will also cover material in any "separate" that is co-published simultaneously with Haworth's special thematic journal issue or DocuSerial. Indexing/abstracting usually covers material at the article/chapter level.
- monographic co-editions are intended for either non-subscribers or libraries which intend to purchase a second copy for their circulating collections.
- monographic co-editions are reported to all jobbers/wholesalers/approval plans. The source journal is listed as the "series" to assist the prevention of duplicate purchasing in the same manner utilized for books-in-series.
- to facilitate user/access services all indexing/abstracting services are encouraged to utilize the co-indexing entry note indicated at the bottom of the first page of each article/chapter/contribution.
- this is intended to assist a library user of any reference tool (whether print, electronic, online, or CD-ROM) to locate the monographic version if the library has purchased this version but not a subscription to the source journal.
- individual articles/chapters in any Haworth publication are also available through the Haworth Document Delivery Service (HDDS).

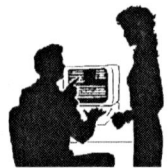

ABOUT THE EDITORS

Andrew Malekoff, MSW, is Associate Executive Director for the North Shore Child and Family Guidance Center in Roslyn Heights, New York, where he has worked since 1977. He is a New York State licensed clinical social worker (LCSW) and credentialed alcoholism and substance abuse counselor (CASAC). Malekoff has been editor of the journal *Social Work with Groups* since 1990. He has taught as an adjunct professor at Adelphi University School of Social Work and is a board member of the Association for the Advancement of Social Work with Groups. Malekoff has written numerous articles, book chapters, essays, narratives, editorials, op-ed pieces, and poetry. Among his nine books and monographs is the critically acclaimed *Group Work with Adolescents: Principles and Practice*, now in its second edition and a main selection of the Behavioral Science Book Club. Malekoff has made presentations across the US and Canada. He is consulting editor for several professional journals and a founder of the Long Island Institute for Group Work with Children and Youth. A former Volunteer in Service to America (VISTA) in Grand Island, Nebraska, Malekoff has also served as Chairman of the City of Long Beach (NY) Civil Service Commission.

Robert Salmon, DSW, is Professor at Hunter College School of Social Work. After joining the faculty in 1971, he later served as Associate Dean or Interim Dean for 16 years. He has been a consulting editor for four social work journals including *Social Work with Groups*. He has presented many papers on social group work practice nationally and internationally. He has published many articles on group work practice and other areas such as work with the aging, drug addiction, and issues in social policy. His most recent book is *Group Work and Aging: Issues in Practice, Research, and Education*, with Roberta Graziano. Two books with Roselle Kurland are *Teaching a Methods Course in Social Work with Groups* and *Group Work Practice in a*

Troubled Society: Problems and Opportunities. He served on the board of directors of the Association for the Advancement of Social Work with Groups for 12 years, including nine years as treasurer of this international organization. He received the Hunter College Award for Excellence in Teaching in 1998. He has received well over 150 grants for the school.

Dominique Moyse Steinberg, DSW, is Assistant Professor at Hunter College School of Social Work, where she has taught as an adjunct professor in the 1980s and 90s. She is chair of the school's division of Group Work Practice. Dr. Steinberg has also been an adjunct faculty member at Smith College and New York University Schools of Social Work. Dr. Steinberg is Founder of The Center for the Advancement of Mutual Aid, based in Vermont and New York. She is author of the books, *The Mutual-Aid Approach to Working With Groups: Helping People Help One Another*, now in its second edition and *The Social Work Student's Research Handbook*. Dr. Steinberg has provided services to various organizations in practice, program design and policy development. These include the New York Family Reception Center, the Child Welfare League of America and the New York Academy for Educational Development, the Children's Defense Fund, Manhattan Teen Pregnancy Network, the Parsons-Sage Institute, Bronx-Lebanon Hospital and the New York Sisters of the Good Shepherd. Dr. Steinberg is an editorial board member of *Social Work with Groups*; a fellow of the Academy of Certified Social Workers; a member, former board member, and former Chair for Endowment for the Association for the Advancement of Social Work with Groups; a member of the NYC/New England chapters of NASW; a former consultant to the NASW Committee on Inquiry; and a professional mediator.

Making Joyful Noise:
The Art, Science,
and Soul of Group Work

CONTENTS

ABOUT THE AUTHORS

Mary C. Bitel, MSW, is Associate Teacher, Tisch School of the Arts, New York University and Adjunct Lecturer, Hunter College School of Social Work. Address correspondence to 26 East 8th Street, Apt. 2A, New York, NY 10003 (mcb12@nyu.edu). Roselle was Mary's professor from 1997-1999. In 2004 Mary entered the PhD program in Social Welfare at Hunter College under the guidance of her mentor and friend.

Lainey Collins, MSW, is Director of Camp Anita Bliss Coler and Off-Season Programs at the Fresh Air Fund, 633 3rd Avenue, New York, NY 10017 (lcollins@freshair.org). Roselle was Lainey's professor and advisor from 1995-1997.

Kris Drumm, MSW, is Executive Director of WolfBear Institute in Wilton Manors, Florida and group work consultant in South Florida. Address correspondence to: 2908 N.W. 6th Terrace, Wilton Manors, FL 33311 (elkedrum@aol.com). Kris knew Roselle at Hunter College where she read the preliminary draft of Kris' paper that appears in this volume.

Helene Ebenstein, MSW, is Coordinator, CAPP Caregiver Resource Center at Mount Sinai Hospital, Mount Sinai Hospital, Box 1252, One Gustave Levy Place, New York, NY 10029 (helene.ebenstein@mountsinai.org). Roselle was Helene's professor in 1997.

Harriet Goodman, DSW, is Associate Professor, Hunter College School of Social Work, 129 East 79th Street, New York, NY 10021 (hgoodman@hunter.cuny.edu). Harriet and Roselle were colleagues at Hunter College School of Social Work for more than 15 years. Roselle encouraged her to design a course to help graduates promote group work in their agencies. The course is the basis for the article presented herein.

Vicki Hallas, BA, is currently a Master of Social Work Student at Hunter College School of Social Work. Address correspondence to 609 West 114th Street, #86, New York, NY 10025 (Vkhallas@aol.com). Roselle was Vicki's professor in 2004 and 2005. She will graduate in 2006.

Priska Imberti, MSW, is a Clinical Social Worker at the North Shore Child and Family Guidance Center, 480 Old Westbury Road, Roslyn Heights, NY and is a school-based social worker (Prixgus@optonline. net). Roselle was Priska's professor from 2001-2003.

Roselle Kurland, PhD, died in June 2005. She was Professor at Hunter College School of Social Work and Co-Editor of *Social Work with Groups* (with Andrew Malekoff) from 1990 until her death in 2005.

Keren Ludwig, MSW, is a Social Worker at The Family Center in Brooklyn, NY. Address correspondence to 463 West Street, #C618, New York, NY 10014 (Kerenmarion@aol.com). Roselle was Keren's professor and academic advisor from 2001-2003.

Andrew Malekoff, MSW, is Associate Director for North Shore Child and Family Guidance Center, 480 Old Westbury Road, Roslyn Heights, NY 11577 and Editor of *Social Work with Groups: A Journal of Community and Clinical Practice* (Anjru@aol.com). Andy and Roselle were Co-Editors of *Social Work with Groups* from 1990-2005.

Helen E. Northen, PhD, died in July, 2006. At the time she was Professor Emerita at the School of Social Work at the University of Southern California. Helen was Roselle's mentor when she attended the School of Social Work at USC. They later became colleagues and friends and co-authors of the third edition of *Social Work with Groups* (Columbia University Press).

Joanna Pudil, MSW, is a Social Worker at Project STAY (Services to Assist Youth), which is affiliated with New York Presbyterian Hospital and Mailman School of Public Health, Columbia University (jlpudil@aol. com). Roselle was Joanna's professor from 2000-2002.

Camille P. Roman, MSW, is in private practice and is an Adjunct Professor at Hunter College School of Social Work. Address correspondence to:

110 East 82nd Street, New York, NY 10028. Camille and Roselle were colleagues and friends for over twenty-five years.

Robert Salmon, DSW, is Professor, Hunter College School of Social Work, 129 East 79th Street, New York, NY 10021 (rssalmon@rcn. com). Roselle and Bob were colleagues at Hunter College School of Social Work and frequent co-presenters, co-authors and co-editors of many keynote addresses, articles, and books.

Dominique Moyse Steinberg, DSW, is Chair, Group Work Practice, Hunter College School of Social Work, 129 East 79th Street, New York, NY 11021 (dmsvt@earthlink.net). Dominique graduated as a groupwork/administration double major in 1982, studied with Roselle in the doctoral program, and eventually became a protégé, close friend, and colleague.

Rachel M. Schneider, MSW, is Clinical Social Worker in private practice and at Memorial Sloan-Kettering Cancer Center, Department of Social Work, 1175 York Avenue, New York, NY 10021 (Rachschneider@aol.com). Roselle was Rachel's professor in 1999.

Sarah Stevenson, MSW, is Senior Trainer, Global Kids, Inc., New York, NY. Address correspondence to: 305 Atlantic Avenue, #2R, Brooklyn, NY 11201 (sarahjoystevenson@hotmail.com). Sarah was a student in Roselle's last seminar class taught at the Hunter College School of Social Work in 2005.

Whitney Wright, MSW, is Founder and Director of Keep It In the Ring, San Francisco, 962 Carolina Street, San Francisco, CA 94107 (whitwright@rcn.com). Roselle was Whitney's professor and academic advisor from 1997-1999.

Foreword

Dr. Roselle Kurland, co-editor with Andrew Malekoff of the journal *Social Work with Groups*, died unexpectedly in early June 2005 at age 62. She had a distinguished career as a practitioner, consultant, editor, author, and professor of social work at Hunter College. She will be long remembered for her many important contributions to the theory and practice of social work with groups.

Dr. Kurland believed in the power of groups when used for social work purposes. Her love of groups became evident when she took her first job as a project specialist with the national program director of the Camp Fire Girls. She participated in developing a demonstration research project on the use of groups for girls with special needs. I was chair of the National Committee, which was composed of volunteers and staff and responsible for such projects. Young as she was, she contributed enthusiasm, skills in interviewing, knowledge of communities, and an ability to work with staff and volunteers as well as with the girls.

At the end of the two-year project, Dr. Kurland decided to get an MSW degree at the University of Southern California where I was a professor. She was an excellent student. Based on her experience with the Camp Fire Girls, she chose to perform her field work in Watts, the most devastated neighborhood in Los Angeles at that time. Her primary assignment, which was evaluated as highly successful, was with a group of adolescent girls and their families. When she presented her work at a public meeting, however, one black man challenged her report, stating that no white woman could help black girls to make it in the white world; and in spite of evidence of her success that challenge followed through the years, resulting in an amazing article that traces her experience and growth in understanding the impact of race and other important factors of difference on her professional competence (*Racial*

[Haworth co-indexing entry note]: "Foreword." Northen, Helen E. Co-published simultaneously in *Social Work with Groups* (The Haworth Press, Inc.) Vol. 29, No. 2/3, 2006, pp. xxxiii-xxxv; and: *Making Joyful Noise: The Art, Science, and Soul of Group Work* (ed: Andrew Malekoff, Robert Salmon, and Dominique Moyse Steinberg) The Haworth Press, Inc., 2006, pp. xxi-xxiii. Single or multiple copies of this article are available for a fee from The Haworth Document Delivery Service [1-800-HAWORTH, 9:00 a.m. - 5:00 p.m. (EST). E-mail address: docdelivery@haworthpress.com].

xxi

Difference and Human Commonality: The Worker-Client Relationship, published in *Social Work with Groups* by The Haworth Press in 2002).

The depth of her understanding of both common and different characteristics and environmental circumstances was essential to her ability to truly accept and respect other clients, colleagues, and friends. Upon graduation, Dr. Kurland returned to her favorite city, New York, to accept a position with the YWCA and later on, with University Settlement.

Deciding that she wanted a career in social work education and supported by a grant from the National Institute of Mental Health, Dr. Kurland eventually returned to USC to work toward a doctoral degree. She majored in advanced practice and research. Her research, based on her former work with the Camp Fire project, was on planning as a process in group development. The findings were based on an in-depth review of the literature and interviews with teachers of group work in graduate schools of social work. Her first published article on this research appeared in the first volume of *Social Work with Groups* published by The Haworth Press in 1978. Further, this work was to serve as a major part of her first monograph, *Group Formation: A Guide to the Development of Successful Groups*, published in 1982 by the School of Social Welfare at the State University of New York, Albany and United Neighborhood Centers of America. She made a significant contribution to the theory and practice of group work.

Upon completing her doctoral program, Dr. Kurland accepted a position at Hunter College School of Social Work, where she happily remained for the rest of her life. Since her doctorate, she made many important contributions to the periodical literature, co-authored at first with George Getzel and later with Andrew Malekoff, Robert Salmon, and others. In 1998, she and Robert Salmon co-authored *Teaching a Methods Course in Social Work With Groups*, published by the Council on Social Work Education. She was my co-author for the latest edition of *Social Work with Groups*, published by Columbia University Press in 2001. What a joy it was to have the benefit of her wisdom and friendship!

Dr. Kurland's published articles on practice with groups are many and include her reflections on the following themes:

1. Formulation of the knowledge and skills involved in planning for new groups.

2. Clarification of major concepts of practice moving from subsequent stages of group development to definition, clarification, illustration, and evaluation.
3. Appropriate use of John Dewey's famous formulation of the problem-solving process with individuals and groups.
4. Understanding the complexity of relationships both among group members and with the worker, including selective concepts from the psychological and social sciences as applied to social work purposes.
5. Depth of understanding of the characteristics of successful social work relationships with individuals, families, and groups and their influence on the success of practice.
6. Perhaps greater than any of these was her focus on the need for self awareness and evaluation of feelings, attitudes, and the ability to be truly helpful to a wide variety of clients whose life experience and social, cultural, and racial factors differ from one's own.

It is clear that Dr. Kurland managed to master the art and science of social relationships, which are the heart of the group.

I hope that future writers and teachers will further formulate the intricacies in the nature and quality of the social worker's role in developing helpful relationships with and among the members of a group. The success of our practice depends upon that. It is clear that Dr. Kurland has mastered the art and science of developing and sustaining professional relationships with clients, colleagues, friends, and significant others. I'm sure that, if she could talk to us today, she might say, with words closely resembling those of Antoine de Saint-Exupéry in *Flight to Arras*: "My love of the group has no need of definition. It is woven of bonds. It is my substance. I am of the group and the group is of me."

Helen E. Northen, PhD
Professor Emerita
University of Southern California

Preface

As we prepared this special collection in tribute to our colleague and friend Roselle Kurland, we received a letter from Helene Ebenstein, one of the contributors. A student in Roselle's *Professional Seminar* class in 1997, Helene remarked that Roselle's impact on her was "enormous." In describing an earlier effort to publish, she remembered how Roselle encouraged her to write: "She forced me to submit the article I wrote to the New York State Society on Aging where it won an award for best paper. They even invited me to Albany to receive the award." She went on, in her letter to us, to recall how Roselle continued to encourage her to write about her group work practice experiences: "She gave me the confidence and tools to continue on the path . . . I guess Roselle was right–I did have something to say."

Ebenstein's remembrance says so much about Roselle the person, Roselle the teacher, and Roselle the missionary for social work with groups. Soon after her untimely death in early June of 2005, the three of us agreed to form a partnership with the purpose of developing a special collection to honor Roselle's legacy. We decided to identify and contact some of Roselle's students and colleagues to contribute, and to ask her mentor Helen Northen to write the foreword to this edition. In our letter of invitation we wrote: "It is our intention that this special issue/book serve to advance social work with groups by highlighting practice, teaching, and writing themes and ideas that were dear to Roselle." We added that we aimed to include scholarly articles as well as shorter, more personal essays.

As the manuscripts trickled in, one by one, leading up to the deadline, our excitement and delight grew. We shared the sentiment that Roselle would have loved this diverse and sometimes "quirky" collection that, as the title suggests, makes joyful noise and captures not only the art and science of group work, but the soul. Perhaps it is the latter, the soul–Roselle's

[Haworth co-indexing entry note]: "Preface." Malekoff, Andrew, Robert Salmon, and Dominique Moyse Steinberg. Co-published simultaneously in *Social Work with Groups* (The Haworth Press, Inc.) Vol. 29, No. 2/3, 2006, pp. xxxvii-xxxix; and: *Making Joyful Noise: The Art, Science, and Soul of Group Work* (ed: Andrew Malekoff, Robert Salmon, and Dominique Moyse Steinberg) The Haworth Press, Inc., 2006, pp. xxv-xxvii. Single or multiple copies of this article are available for a fee from The Haworth Document Delivery Service [1-800-HAWORTH, 9:00 a.m. - 5:00 p.m. (EST). E-mail address: docdelivery@haworth press.com].

Available online at http://www.haworthpress.com/web/SWG
xxv

soul–that one feels most strongly in pouring through the pages of this special collection. It is as if our collective voice is saying to Roselle, "See what you taught us? Don't worry. We will keep your voice alive, here and there and everywhere"; and to the readers, "You really need to get to know Roselle. She was a real character. She had great intellect, great humor, and great soul. And, she was bold."

This diverse collection is a combination of the personal and the professional. It includes articles that emerged from keynote addresses that were first presented by Kurland and Salmon at symposia of the Association for the Advancement of Social Work with Groups: on *making joyful noise* through group work and on understanding the special qualities and world view of those drawn to group work.

The collection includes articles with themes that represent some of the key phrases of Roselle's mantra: "Stay in the mess" (Hallas) and "Be Bold" (Ludwig and Imberti), and "What is the purpose?" (Kurland and Salmon), a mantra that is reinforced in a piece dedicated to preserving and promoting the essential power of group work in its "undiluted entirety" (Drumm).

The articles cover a range of age groups, diverse populations and unique settings and include wonderful illustrations on the use of activity and discussion in groups: a classroom-based poetry club for young children (Malekoff), the meaning of camp for preadolescents (Collins), boxing group for adolescents living in the inner city (Wright), self-defense classes for adults (Stevenson), and caregiver support groups for the elderly (Ebenstein).

And, what would a collection dedicated to Roselle be without stepping into the classroom and promoting scholarship: understanding the art, science, heart and ethics of teaching social group work (Moyse Steinberg); advancing the education of advanced group work practitioners (Goodman); revisiting Kurland and Salmon's book, *Teaching a Methods Course in Social Work with Groups* (Bitel); and presenting guidelines to encourage practitioners (and others) to write about group work (Malekoff).

Although we encouraged contributors to choose their own themes to write about, it was inevitable that separation, loss and endings would find their place in this special collection: group bereavement support group for spouses (Schneider), how a group can survive when its leader takes a leave of absence (Pudil), and a worker's personal grief and its impact on processing a group's termination (Roman).

After months of reviewing manuscripts, communicating by phone and email, and working separately with authors to revise their work, the three of us approached the date that we agreed to get together at Hunter College School of Social Work to review the complete collection.

December 20, 2005, our scheduled meeting date, turned out to be the second day of the transit strike that paralyzed New York City for three days. We each found our separate ways through the maze of grid-locked streets and endless parade of pedestrians walking shoulder-to-shoulder en route to work. Without planning a "pre-group" destination, we ended up together at the same "greasy spoon" around the corner from Hunter on Lexington Avenue. Malekoff was the first to arrive and was sitting at the counter eating a cheddar cheese omelet; next came Moyse Steinberg who ordered coffee, and then came Salmon who asked for coffee and a slice of pound cake. It was a place that Kurland used to frequent, once upon a time.

We welcome you to this special collection, a blend of writings and reflections by practitioners and academics; students, colleagues, and friends of Roselle Kurland. For those of you who didn't know her, we hope that you will get to know Roselle through the essays and articles presented herein. Most importantly, though, it is our aim that this volume will inspire your practice, teaching, and supervision and provide you with some of the tools necessary to become missionaries who will continue to spread the message about social work with groups.

Andrew Malekoff
Robert Salmon
Dominique Moyse Steinberg
Editors

Making Joyful Noise:
Presenting, Promoting, and Portraying
Group Work to and for the Profession

Roselle Kurland
Robert Salmon

SUMMARY. This article advocates for better articulating the value and uniqueness of group work, developing hard evidence to demonstrate that the paucity of group work education and training is a serious problem, and developing scholars and teachers of group work who will write and speak about the distinctiveness of group work as a positive, optimistic, empowering and affirming way of working with people. *[Article copies available for a fee from The Haworth Document Delivery Service: 1-800-HAWORTH. E-mail address: <docdelivery@haworthpress.com> Website: <http://www.HaworthPress.com> © 2006 by The Haworth Press, Inc. All rights reserved.]*

KEYWORDS. Group work, group work education, group work scholarship, group work training

Originally published in 1996, in B. Stempler and M. Glass (eds.), *Social Group Work Today and Tomorrow: Moving from Theory to Advanced Training and Practice*, 19-32.

Reprinted with an introduction by Robert Salmon.

[Haworth co-indexing entry note]: "Making Joyful Noise: Presenting, Promoting, and Portraying Group Work to and for the Profession." Kurland, Roselle, and Robert Salmon. Co-published simultaneously in *Social Work with Groups* (The Haworth Press, Inc.) Vol. 29, No. 2/3, 2006, pp. 1-15; and: *Making Joyful Noise: The Art, Science, and Soul of Group Work* (ed: Andrew Malekoff, Robert Salmon, and Dominique Moyse Steinberg) The Haworth Press, Inc., 2006, pp. 1-15. Single or multiple copies of this article are available for a fee from The Haworth Document Delivery Service [1-800-HAWORTH, 9:00 a.m. - 5:00 p.m. (EST). E-mail address: docdelivery@haworthpress.com].

INTRODUCTION

Making Joyful Noise . . . , the first three words in the title of this book, seemed a fitting choice for a publication prepared as a tribute to Roselle Kurland. Roselle and I previously used them in the title of our Plenary Presentation at the Fourteenth Annual Symposium of AASWG in 1992 (published in Stempler, B., and Glass, M., 1996), which is reprinted here.

The idea for the article was given to us by Ruth Middleman, who said, "Let us be noisy" in support of our beloved practice method, social work with groups (Middleman, R., 1990). She urged us all to use everything possible–talent, skill, knowledge, humor, and persistence–to protect and preserve good group work practice. Roselle took this advice to heart, and it was reflected upon, again, in two subsequent published Plenary Presentations about group work's battle to survive (Kurland, R., and Salmon, R., 2004, and In Press, 2006). The battle is needed. Andrew Malekoff (Malekoff, A., 2004) reflected on the problem in his poem, "My Kind of Group Work (GW)" when he wrote:

> *It's the GW that is a rare gem in the human services, yet faces extinction.*

The problems discussed in this reprinted article have been with us for a long time. Emmanual Tropp in a remarkably prescient article in the first issue of *Social Work with Groups*, titled "Whatever Happened to Group Work," discussed the very same educational and practice issues we face today, almost 30 years later (Tropp, E., 1978). In his article, he ended with an expression of hope for the future. We maintain that hope, but also strive to enlist group work practitioners to join in the efforts to help the method flourish. The message delivered in the articles by Tropp, by Middleman, by Kurland and Salmon, and others as well, is captured in the final lines of Malekoff's poem:

> *It's the GW that needs workers to stay the course*
> *administrators to support the way*
> *and missionaries to spread the word.*

Robert Salmon

REFERENCES

Kurland, R. and Salmon, R. (1996). Making Joyful Noise: Presenting, Promoting, and Portraying Group Work to and for the Profession. In B.Stempler and M. Glass (Eds.) *Social Group Work Today and Tomorrow: Moving from Theory to Advanced Training and Practice*. New York: The Haworth Press, Inc., pp. 19-32.

Kurland, R. and Salmon, R. (in press-2007). Caught in the Doorway Between Education and Practice: Group Work's Battle for Survival. In C. Cohen, M. Phillips and M. Hansen (Eds.) *Think Group: Strength and Diversity through Group Work*. New York: The Haworth Press, Inc.

Kurland, R. and Salmon, R. with M. Bitel, H. Goodman, K. Ludwig, E.W. Newman and N. Sullivan. (2004). The survival of Social Group Work: A Call to Action. *Social Work with Groups*, 27 (1), 3-16.

Malekoff, A. (2004). Poem: My Kind of Group Work (GW). In *Group Work with Adolescents: Principles and Practice*, 2nd edition, New York: The Guilford Press, p. 37.

Middleman, R.(1990). Group Work and The Heimlich Maneuver: Unchoking Social Work Education. Plenary Presentation, 12th Annual Symposium of the Association for the Advancement of Social Work with Groups. Miami, Florida, p. 37.

Tropp, E. (1978). Whatever Happened to Group Work? *Social Work with Groups*, 1 (1), 85-94.

"Once more unto the breach, dear friends, once more; or close the wall up with our English dead!" (Shakespeare, *King Henry the Fifth*, act 3, scene 1, line 2). Does that sound familiar? Does the half-remembered line stir you a bit? It should as that surely was the intention of the author. Shakespeare gave Henry this line as the start of a powerful speech whose purpose was to rouse his vastly outnumbered forces to battle the French. His were the weapons of war of his time, as well as glorious language, and an appeal to courage.

The analogy to Henry is intentional. As we gather here today, we need to understand that we too are a vastly outnumbered force in a battle of a different kind. It *is* a battle–not bloody, but nevertheless intense–to preserve social work with groups as a viable part of social work practice today. The tools we use are not the symbolic primitive weapons of physical warfare. Ours are different. We need to use our knowledge of systems, of groups, and of individuals to preserve what we feel is important. These attributes, as well as organizational skills, and the ". . . use of humor and fun, playfulness along with planfulness in (our) practice approaches" (Middleman, 1990) are what we have to protect our method.

It needs protection. In a sobering research paper presented earlier this year, Martin Birnbaum and Charles Auerbach asked their au-

dience to imagine a situation where social work students graduated without course work and field experience in work with
individuals. The suggestion was inconceivable, but sadly it is often reality for group work. Most students are graduating without a
group course and group work field experience and *are* likely to be
practicing with groups. The irony is that work with groups is a major component of social work practice while graduate education
has practically eliminated group work as a specialized area of
study. (Birnbaum and Auerbach, 1992)

Two years ago, in a plenary address at the Twelfth Annual Symposium in Miami, Ruth R. Middleman delivered a call to action to those
concerned with the place of group work in our profession. "Let us be
noisy," she said.

Let us be watchdogs and whistle-blowers at omissions and mis-
representations concerning group work in our social work publications. Let us write interpretive statements about the breadth of
group work, letters to the editors of journals, letters to the Educational Planning Commission of Council on Social Work Education
and the Program Committee of the National Association of Social
Workers (NASW), editorials for journals where we have influence. Let us accent an influence on the profession-at-large, sending our scholarship beyond the group journals. We must do our
homework to prepare conceptual, scholarly, clarifying papers on
social work with groups and provide interior views of our practice
to others. (Middleman, 1990)

In this chapter, we build on Middleman's call to action to look at
group work's current situation within the social work profession and
consider strategies to present, promote, and portray group work to and
for the profession.

It is almost sixty years since Wilbur Newstetter articulated the first
definition of social group work (Newstetter, 1935), and yet many in our
profession do not really understand or appreciate group work. That lack
of understanding was also present in group work's preprofessional days
before the 1930s when the majority of group workers worked in settlement houses, Y's, youth organizations, and playground and recreation
departments (Wenocur and Reisch, 1989), *and* when the main focus of
their work was on the well rather than the mentally ill. As Gertrude Wilson described it in 1937, group workers and caseworkers had little pro-

fessional contact. She depicted a situation of mutual exclusiveness caused by indifference and latent antagonism characterized by only intermittent cooperation.

> The problem of acceptance by other social work practitioners was felt by many group workers. The scorn exhibited toward "those workers who play with children," "run dances," "go camping," or "teach arts and crafts" is well remembered. In 1936 it was reported that the California Conference of Social Work seriously questioned whether group workers were social workers. Faculty members of the School of Social Service Administration of the University of Chicago minced no words in their exclusion of any study of an activity remotely connected with recreation. The general population of the country was still dominated by the "Protestant ethic." (Wilson, 1976)

Unfortunately, the lack of understanding of group work has not changed very much. Just three years ago, we invited ten outstanding alumni who had majored in group work at Hunter College School of Social Work to participate in a panel discussion. We asked them to identify what they thought were the most important things they had gained from their group work courses at Hunter and what they had not gotten, and what they wished they had because they realized now that they needed it. Almost to a person, what these alumni identified as needed was the ability to explain group work to others–to colleagues, supervisors, supervisees, professionals of other disciplines, and funding sources. They told of incidents and attitudes in their agencies that illustrated that group work was not well understood by professionals–social workers and others–with whom they came into contact. Said one graduate, a social worker in a hospital:

> I was surprised to find that very few people know about group work, that there can be psychologists, psychiatrists, and social workers, too, who just think that social group work is casework in a group. You just throw the group together and talk to each person, and you control everything, and then that's fine, you have started a group. . . . The other thing that I found surprising is how much group work is looked down upon. It's not acknowledged as an actual training with its own theories and its own skills. . . . It has been a struggle for me to communicate to other disciplines that social

workers *do* know something about running groups. (Cavrell-Epstein, 1989)

Another graduate, a social worker in a community mental health clinic, lamented that other social workers in his agency seemed to have little understanding of or appreciation for work with groups. "They do not really think that the work that I do with clients is important," he said. "It's individual therapy that they view as the real work, not group work" (Munoz, 1989). And still another graduate, a director of a small agency working with youth, said she struggled to explain group work to representatives of foundations and other funding sources. "When funders make a site visit and come into a room and see the kids working on a project together and maybe it seems chaotic, how do you explain that what's going on is important, that there's more to it than meets the eye?" she asked (Lyons, 1989).

Underlying the difficulty in explaining group work to others in social work, we believe, is a lack of respect that many, though certainly not all, in our profession hold toward group work. That lack of respect is difficult to combat, for often it is not expressed directly. Group work is *said* to be respected, but beneath the surface lurks attitudes that assert: "If you know how to work with individuals, then you can work with a group for group work is simply casework multiplied," or "Group work is superficial. It's only in individual work where there is true depth," or "Activities, so often used by group workers, aren't really helpful. The psychological insights that stem from discussion of problems are what matter."

We have faced these attitudes toward group work throughout our history. Group work's use of activities, for instance, has been causing professional discomfort for sixty years or more. The early group workers who moved into social work from recreation and leisure-time programs were viewed with skepticism then and questions about whether they really were social workers (Middleman, 1982). For many social workers, that is not so different today.

After much "lobbying" on her part a second-year social work student, whose placement was at a large state hospital for the mentally ill, convinced the director of in-patient services to allow her to form and lead a singing group. Her supervisor's attitude toward her work with the singing group was made quite evident when she told the student, "Do not bother to write process recordings on the singing group. We don't have to talk much about that group. Just do process for your therapy group."

Many in social work, even today, do not understand or appreciate the value of activity in group work practice. They are much more at ease with and accord higher status and legitimacy to group work practice that uses words exclusively. Helen Harris Perlman, reviewing changes in the first decade of the NASW, 1955-1965, sounded almost relieved when she wrote about group work.

> It has burst the too narrow seams of its basketball uniform and arts-and-crafts smocks; increasingly it appears in the contrasting symbolic garments that bespeak the poles of its present scope–the authority–cool white coats of hospital and clinical personnel and the play-it-cool windbreaker of the street-corner gang worker . . . group work is increasingly involved with the persons, places, problems and even some of the processes that not too long ago were assumed to 'belong' to case work. (Perlman, 1965)

Greatly contributing to the misconceptions that social workers have about group work and the need to explain our method to our colleagues in social work is the current state of graduate social work education. The paucity of curriculum content on work with groups and the causes of that vacuum have been described in papers and plenary addresses at past symposia (Birnbaum, 1990; Middleman, 1990; Parry, 1991).

These presentations have made us aware that, from the 1960s on, the CSWE moved toward curriculum standards that required schools of social work to emphasize the *generic* in social work practice. The move was intended to define more sharply social work's identity as one profession. That effort, however, has been a disaster for group work. Left out and rapidly disappearing from our profession are the *specific* beliefs, knowledge, and skills that are the hallmark of group work.

Because group workers were always a small minority of social work faculty, generic practice courses, by necessity, were taught largely by persons whose expertise was in work with individuals and who had little or no social group work experience. The emphasis in such courses was on either work with individuals or on a kind of group work that focuses on individual group members to the neglect of the group, or on the individual and the psychological to the neglect of the social.

Given the growing neglect of group work in graduate social work education for close to three decades, it is no wonder that our graduates cry out that their colleagues do not understand, appreciate, or respect group work. It is no wonder that they have difficulty explaining it.

So where do we go from here? What are the implications for action of group work's current situation? What do we need to do to present, promote, and portray group work to and for the profession? How can we go about making joyful noise? We recommend seven directions that our efforts must take.

First, we ourselves must get better at articulating the value and uniqueness of group work's approach to (and emphasis in) working with people. The humanistic views that undergird our work, the need of people for acceptance, for belonging, and for group membership, the quest for social justice and for social change, for consciousness-raising and empowerment–all of these have been spoken and written about with conviction and eloquence by participants in past symposia[1] and all are vital to an identification of group work's uniqueness and importance. What remains pivotal, as well, to an articulation of the uniqueness and specialness of group work is the concept of mutual aid, described first by Peter Kropotkin (1914) and made central to group work by William Schwartz (1971). The process of mutual aid really is unique to social group work. We need to get better at identifying its importance and depicting what mutual aid looks like in group work practice.

In a previous publication (Kurland and Salmon, 1992), the authors attempted to do this by discussing the major differences between group work and casework in a group. In fact, *casework in a group* can be defined as practice that does not maximize mutual aid among group members. Casework in a group is mutual aid-less! It can be seen when a worker views each member only as an individual and applies individual personality theories and dynamics without appreciating or understanding the impact of such group concepts as size, roles, norms, communication patterns, member interaction and influence, and group stages, to name but a few. Similarly, casework in a group is being practiced when a worker allots time to each individual group member, in turn, to talk about progress on issues of concern or when a worker allots time in round-robin fashion and does not maximize group interaction.

Group work, on the other hand, can be defined as a process where mutual aid is central and maximized. In such group work practice, the situation, problem, or need of one group member provides an opportunity for *all* in the group to examine their own situations, problems, or needs as they draw upon their own experiences to respond to their fellow members. Merely jumping in to give advice to another member is *not* group work. In fact, it is the quality of the *mutual* aid process that occurs in a group that is central in distinguishing social group work practice from other group efforts. We need to talk about the mutual aid process more, and more clearly, as we attempt to describe group work to others.

Second, we need to develop data to support our claim that the lack of group work education and training matters. The reality that many groups are being led today by workers untrained in social group work practice has been identified previously as problematic (Birnbaum, Middleman, and Huber, 1989). But we need to do more than bemoan that fact. We need to be able to identify what difference that makes. We need evidence.

A recently completed research study by Dominique Moyse Steinberg (1992) is an important step in providing some of the evidence we need. Steinberg interviewed some 30 social workers who were working with groups, half of whom had substantial graduate social work education in group work and half of whom had minimal or no group work education or training. She spoke with them in depth about their practice with groups and found important differences between those with group work education and those without it.

There were differences in the way these workers conceptualized the group, exercised control, and viewed their role and their use of self. Those without education in group work tended to see the group as a place for individual change within a supportive environment. They tended to play a central role throughout the group's life, to direct many of their interventions to individual group members, and to assume a great deal of control. Those with group work education expected the group members to integrally affect and effect the shape and movement of the group. They saw group purpose as central. They tended to direct many of their interventions and expectations to the group as a whole and to be aware of the impact the stages of group development had over time on their role and their use of themselves.

Especially important were differences regarding conflict held by these workers. While those with group work education expected conflict to occur as a natural result of group life and viewed conflict as opportunity for important work in the group, those without education in group work tended to regard conflict as an intrusion into the group's affairs, an unwelcome interruption, a threat to the group, and a hurdle that needed to be quickly resolved so that the group could move on.

Steinberg's findings are important. They tell us that group work education really does matter and that who leads a group makes a difference in the quality of professional practice. They provide us with the kind of evidence that we need to argue for greater attention to group work in social work education and agency supervision and training. They provide much direction for future efforts and research. We need more such work to use in our attempts to substantiate the importance of group work education.

Third, we need to present both our articulation of group work's uniqueness and importance and our evidence that group work education and training make a difference to a wide range of people–to students and supervisees, to colleagues, to agency supervisors and administrators, to social work faculty members, to deans and directors of schools of social work, to CSWE, to NASW.

Our efforts to establish group work's place in both education and practice need to go in two directions simultaneously. From the bottom up, our students, supervisees, and colleagues in agencies and on faculties might well be helped to become ambassadors, even missionaries perhaps, for the practice and teaching of group work where it is needed. From the top down, our deans and administrators, and our national organizations need to be helped to see that group work is endangered. They must be held accountable for ensuring that social group work is not allowed to disappear.

The efforts of AASWG and many of its members to influence CSWE's curriculum policy statements, establish a presence on its policy-making boards, and open lines of communication and collaboration with NASW certainly are steps in this direction. We must continue to make our presence known with ever-increasing vigor and be both reactive and proactive as we engage with our national social work organizations.

Fourth, we, ourselves, must become involved in agency training, consultation, and supervision. We need to use our beliefs and passion about the importance of group work, our knowledge and our skills to enhance workers' understanding, appreciation, and respect for groups and group work practice, and to improve their skill in group leadership.

We need to go out of our way to be responsive to calls for help from agencies and practitioners who are interested in work with groups.

> Five years ago at the tenth annual symposium in Baltimore, I was approached by two young individuals from Iowa whom I did not know. Would I be willing to supervise them around their work with groups of teenagers who had been sexually abused, they wanted to know. They had tried to obtain supervision from staff at the agency where they were leading groups, as well as from professionals outside the agency, but were unable to find anyone with expertise in social group work. They had even looked for courses

on group work that they might take. To put it mildly, I was surprised at their request. How would this work, I wanted to know. They suggested telephone supervision once a month. I had my doubts. But their earnestness, the initiative they took in approaching me, their commitment to their work, and their desire for help were impossible to disregard.

I agreed and thus began one of the most unusual and rewarding professional relationships I have experienced. We spoke on the phone for an hour or more once a month for over a year until their work with teens ended. Each month we had to make sure we had the time straight for our calls– "O.K., seven o'clock your time, that's eight o'clock my time." The conversations were fun and exciting. They directed our conversations with questions and concerns that they had and the situations they described. Often, they challenged my responses–"But why are you suggesting that? Could you say more about what you mean?"–and made *me* really think. Our common interest in the work united us even when we hardly knew each other and could not even talk face-to-face. We all benefited. (Kurland, 1992)

There is a real thirst for knowledge about groups out there and we need to respond to it in creative ways. We need to share our expertise in work with groups, to make it available to others.

One special group with which we need to work is field instructors to help them supervise students around work with groups. Another might be faculty members who want to expand their knowledge. Our efforts need to be aimed to help both agency staff and faculty understand that it is in their interest and that of their clients and students to move to the inclusion and/or expansion of groups (Kurland, Getzel, and Salmon, 1986).

Fifth, we need to continue to talk to ourselves. Doing so strengthens our ability to then go out and talk to others. At these symposia, in the local chapters of AASWG, and through the journal, *Social Work with Groups*, we find our voice and our song and revitalize and energize ourselves.

If history is instructive, then we can learn from the past that we need a place of our own within a social work profession where work with individuals predominates. A place where we can share our ideas, and practice with others with similar interests and experiences. The formation of the AASWG in 1979 came as a response to such a need, just as in 1946 group workers felt it was necessary to form their own organization, the American Association of Group Workers (Wenocur and Reisch, 1989).

Sixth, we need to develop our scholarship and write and speak about our work in special group work forums such as the journal *Social Work with Groups*, these symposia, and the group work section of CSWE's annual program meeting. Additionally, we must also present our work in the forums of our profession throughout its many journals and conferences.

> Last spring we submitted an abstract for a paper we wished to present at the annual program meeting of CSWE. We purposely did *not* submit it as part of the specialized group work section, for we wanted to speak to a wider audience. Much to our surprise, we received a call from one of the professional staff at the Council. Wanting to be helpful, she asked whether we had made a mistake. Since the words "group work" were in the abstract's title, she wondered whether we meant to submit it to the special group work section. When we told her that no mistake had been made, she said that it certainly was possible to consider our abstract a general submission.

We do ourselves a disservice when we talk *only* to each other. We need to present our ideas and our work to a diverse social work audience if that work is to have impact and influence. We cannot allow others to isolate our work and our ideas and we cannot isolate ourselves.

Too often, our presentations and papers just describe our work with groups. Though description of our work is important, it is not enough. Our scholarship needs to bring together the doing and the thinking of group work practice. Descriptions of practice need to be examined conceptually, critically, analytically. Presentations of work with groups will be strengthened and made more useful if description is linked to theory. In an editorial in *Social Work with Groups*, the editors (Roselle Kurland and Andrew Malekoff, 1992) discuss the kinds of articles they would like to see submitted to the journal. They note, "In articles that portray practice through the presentation of descriptive vignettes and examples, the rationale that underpins the practice, the thinking behind it, and the implications for future practice with groups are crucial elements" (Kurland and Malekoff, 1992).

Seventh, we need to begin to encourage and develop the scholars and teachers of group work's future. When we encounter workers with interest in and passion for work with groups, we should ask whether they have considered teaching, be it on a full-time basis or as adjunct instructors. We need to make ourselves available as mentors for such persons and support their efforts to engage in the teaching and training of new social workers. Those with conviction about and commitment to group work need to become a force and a presence on social work faculties. To do so, they will need to develop well-rounded expertise in areas beyond group work. Then, as they teach courses, such as human behavior, research, and practice and policy, in addition to specialized courses in group work, they will bring their sensitivity and understanding of groups and group work practice to those courses. They will have an impact.

The actions that we are recommending to present, promote, and portray group work are really not so very new. There are no miraculous elixirs; hard work is required of us. We have tried to be very practical and quite specific in delineating what we must do. In summary, we propose seven areas on which to focus our energy.

- We need to get better at articulating the value and uniqueness of group work.
- We need to develop hard evidence to demonstrate that the paucity of group work education and training is a problem.
- We need to widely disseminate both our articulation and our evidence.
- We need to get involved in agency training, consultation, and supervision.
- We need to continue to talk to ourselves.
- We need to develop our scholarship and write and speak about our work in specialized group work forums as well as in the wider forums of the social work profession.
- We need to encourage and develop the scholars and teachers of group work's future.

Social group work is a very positive and optimistic way of working with people. It is truly empowering. It is truly affirming of people's strengths. It is a fact that the very act of forming a group is a statement of belief in people's strengths, a statement of belief that everyone has something to give to others. In today's troubled world, real group work is needed more than ever. We cannot let it disappear. We truly must make joyful noise.

NOTE

1. See, for example, Urania Glassman and Len Kates, *Group Work: A Humanistic Approach*, Sage Publications, 1990, Hans Falck, *Social Work: The Membership Perspective*, New York: Springer Publishing Company, 1988, Margot Breton, Learning from Social Group Work Traditions, Proceedings, 11th Annual Symposium on Social Work with Groups, Montreal, 1989.

REFERENCES

Birnbaum, Martin. (1990, October). "Group Work, the Spotted Owl: An Endangered Species in Social Work Education." Presented at the 12th Annual Symposium on Social Work with Groups, Miami, Florida.

Birnbaum, Martin, Middleman, Ruth, and Huber, Ruth. (1989). "Where Social Workers Obtain Their Knowledge Base in Group Work." Presented at the Annual Meeting of NASW.

Birnbaum, Martin and Auerbach, Charles. (1992, March). "Group Work in Graduate Social Work Education–The Price of Neglect." Presented at the Council on Social Work Education Annual Program meeting, Kansas City, Kansas.

Breton, Margot. (1989, October). "Learning from Social Group Work Traditions." Proceedings of the Eleventh Annual Symposium on Social Work with Groups, Montreal, Canada.

Cavrell-Epstein, Dawn. (1989). Panel discussion. Hunter College School of Social Work, New York, New York, November 9.

Falck, Hans. (1988). *Social Work: The Membership Perspective*. New York: Springer Publishing Company.

Glassman, Urania and Kates, Len. (1990). *Group Work: A Humanistic Approach*. Sage Publications, Inc., Newbury Park, CA.

Kropotkin, Peter. (1914). *Mutual Aid: A Factor of Evolution*. Reissued in 1989 by Black Rose Books: Montreal, Canada.

Kurland, Roselle. (1992, September). Personal statement to class at Hunter College School of Social Work.

Kurland, Roselle, Getzel, George, and Salmon, Robert. (1986). "Sowing Groups in Infertile Fields: Curriculum and Other Strategies to Overcome Resistance to the Formation of New Groups." In *Innovations in Social Work: Feedback From Practice to Theory*, Marvin Parnes (Ed.). New York: The Haworth Press, Inc.

Kurland, Roselle and Malekoff, Andrew. (1992). Editorial. *Social Work with Groups*, Vol. 15, No. 4, pp. 1-2.

Kurland, Roselle and Salmon, Robert. (1992). "Group Work vs. Casework in a Group: Principles and Implications for Teaching and Practice." *Social Work with Groups*, Vol. 15, No. 4, pp. 3-14.

Lyons, Eileen. (1989). Panel discussion. Hunter College School of Social Work, New York, New York, November 9.

Middleman, Ruth. (1982). *The Non-Verbal Method in Working with Groups*, enlarged edition. Hebron, CT: Practitioners' Press.

Middleman, Ruth. (1990, October). "Group Work and the Heimlich Maneuver: Unchoking Social Work Education." Plenary Address, 12th Annual Symposium on Social Work with Groups, Miami, Florida.

Munoz, Manuel. (1989). Panel discussion. Hunter College School of Social Work, New York, New York, November 9.

Newstetter, Wilbur. (1935). "What is Social Group Work?" *Proceedings of the National Conference of Social Work*, pp. 291-299. New York: National Conference of Social Work.

Parry, Joan. (1991, October). Plenary Address, 13th Annual Symposium on Social Work with Groups, Akron, Ohio.

Perlman, Helen Harris. (1965). "Social Work Method: A Review of the Past Decade."*Social Work*, Vol. X, No. 4.

Schwartz, William and Zalba, Serapio. (1971). *The Practice of Group Work*. New York: Columbia University Press.

Shakespeare, William. *King Henry the Fifth*, III, I, 2.

Steinberg, Dominique Moyse. (1992). *The Impact of Group Work Education on Social Work Practitioners' Work with Groups*. Doctoral dissertation, City University of New York, New York.

Wenocur, Stanley and Reisch, Michael. (1989). *From Charity to Enterprise: The Development of Social Work in a Market Economy*. Urbana: University of Illinois Press.

Wilson, Gertrude. (1976). From Practice to Theory: A Personalized History. In *Theories of Social Work with Groups*. Robert Roberts and Helen Northen (Eds.). New York: Columbia University Press.

The Essential Power of Group Work

Kris Drumm

SUMMARY. For almost two decades, leaders in the field of social group work have been warning that the foundational principles and practice of group work as a modality are in danger of being absorbed into generalist social work practice. This paper expands upon the appeal of leaders in the social group work field to generate an environment in which group work is recognized as an integral method in social work practice and education. This paper examines group work as a powerful methodology in social work practice with a specific theoretical framework and skill base that is fundamental to the social work profession. The characteristics of group work's strengths are explored with a comprehensive overview that inspires renewed commitment to preserving, practicing and promoting social group work as a viable and integral part of social work practice. *[Article copies available for a fee from The Haworth Document Delivery Service: 1-800-HAWORTH. E-mail address: <docdelivery@haworthpress.com> Website: <http://www.HaworthPress.com> © 2006 by The Haworth Press, Inc. All rights reserved.]*

KEYWORDS. Social group work, mutual aid, stage management, social work curricula, Maslow's Hierarchy of Needs

INTRODUCTION

For the past fifteen years Kurland and Salmon (1992, 1996, 2002, 2004) along with Middleman (1990) have been warning practitioners

[Haworth co-indexing entry note]: "The Essential Power of Group Work." Drumm, Kris. Co-published simultaneously in *Social Work with Groups* (The Haworth Press, Inc.) Vol. 29, No. 2/3, 2006, pp. 17-31; and: *Making Joyful Noise: The Art, Science, and Soul of Group Work* (ed: Andrew Malekoff, Robert Salmon, and Dominique Moyse Steinberg) The Haworth Press, Inc., 2006, pp. 17-31. Single or multiple copies of this article are available for a fee from The Haworth Document Delivery Service [1-800-HAWORTH, 9:00 a.m. - 5:00 p.m. (EST). E-mail address: docdelivery@haworthpress.com].

that social group work theory, principles and practice are in danger of being absorbed and dispersed into the greater social work field as generalist practice becomes the current predominant approach to services and to social work education. In three separate addresses to the Annual Symposium of the Association for the Advancement of Social Work with Groups (AASWG), Kurland and Salmon (1992, 2002, 2004) appealed to social group workers to strategize to create an environment in which group work is honored in its right as an integral method in social work practice and education. Middleman (1990, p. 30) made a call for action fifteen years ago, beseeching group workers to go forth and "be noisy" articulating our understanding of the values and knowledge of group work. Kurland and Salmon call for a "Joyful Noise" about group work (1992, 1996).

This paper seeks to be loud and clear about the reasons group work is a powerful method with a specific theoretical framework and skill base that is fundamental to the social work profession. The components of group work's strengths are presented with the intention of providing practitioners and agencies with a comprehensive overview that inspires renewed commitment to preserving, practicing and promoting social group work in its undiluted entirety.

THE DECLINE OF SOCIAL GROUP WORK EDUCATION AND PRACTICE

There is an abundance of literature on the principles and efficacy of social work with groups (Cohen, 1995; Dies, 1995; Garvin, 2001; Getzel, 2003; Gitterman, 2003; Kurland and Salmon, 1992; Middleman and Wood, 1990; Northen and Kurland, 2001; Shulman, 1999). Nevertheless, there is a continuing omission of comprehensive group work curricula (Birnbaum and Auerbach, 1994; Steinberg, 2002).

The decline of social work education in group work began in 1969 when the Council on Social Work Education (CSWE) decided to integrate casework, community organizing, and group work into one generalist method (Kurland and Salmon, 2002; Magen, 1998). The percentage of social work graduate programs that had concentrations in the group work method went from 76% in 1963 to 22% in 1981, and in a 1992 survey of graduate schools of social work, the percentage had dropped to an alarming seven percent (Birnbaum and Auerbach, 1992). The continuous diminishing of group work's importance as a specialized modality in foundational curricula relegates the methodology to a status that appears to be regarded as peripheral to social work practice.

The decrease in social group work visibility and presence in social work curricula may have led to fewer social workers who view group work as an effective response to client needs (Cohen, 1995). As a result, group work is frequently marginalized as non-essential and less serious and substantive than casework (Kurland and Salmon, 1992; Cohen, 1995). The marginalization of social group work within the social work profession may indicate a fundamental flaw in the perception and perspective on where social group work exists in relation to casework, community organizing and administration.

Social group work challenges the dominant political sensibilities of individualism, competition, dualism, and authoritarianism. The exclusion of social group work curricula and the dilution and distortions of group work theory and practice may be reflecting the current political climate, policy, and national events, all of which impact social work (Middleman, 1990).

Social workers who are group workers struggle with agencies to legitimize and include social group work as a crucial method of practice. This struggle for legitimacy parallels the struggles that many of our disenfranchised clients face. Ironically it also parallels the struggle that the social work field has faced since the early nineteen hundreds when Flexner (1915) publicly posed the question whether social work was a profession.

PRINCIPLE POWER

At the 2005 Annual Symposium of the Association for the Advancement of Social Work with Groups (AASWG), Dominique Moyse Steinberg eloquently referred to the "magic" of group work in her tribute to the legacy of Roselle Kurland. The magic she is referring to is the power that is created by skillful practitioners who adhere to the basic precepts of social work with groups. Social group work principles, theory, and skill bases formulate a powerful potion for spelling and dispelling the forces that obstruct the growth and freedom of the people we work with, our agencies and ourselves.

These elements of social group work are remarkably effective when combined and practiced in the cauldron of the contemporary social work milieu. The resulting "brew" benefits and enhances not only the individual participants' social functionality but the agency's functionality as well. Conscientiously practiced social group work improves all of the systems it is practiced in and the synergy of the systems as well.

Group work requires workers to bring the underlying and hidden issues and feelings to the surface in a public way (Shulman, 1998). Middleman (1990, p. 24) states, "it takes guts to work with individuals while others watch what you do." Breaking taboos such as talking about sexuality or abuse in front of others deviates from societal norms. The exposed nature of social work groups' reciprocal exchange is outside the boundaries of our individualistic and dualistic conditioning. The ability to shatter false dichotomies is a skill of the adept group worker who facilitates a process that bursts the bounds of teacher-student, doctor-patient, parent-child power dyads (Shulman and Gitterman, 2003).

Social group work has been characterized as being in the swamp, or the muck, or the mess (Schon, 1987) because it embraces the get down and dirty of relating and struggling with problems in meaningful ways (Kurland and Salmon, 1992). Truth and conflicts are brought to the surface and participants are guided to examine and grapple with all of the positions and options involved.

Practitioners are required to be able to be vulnerable and flexible and able to take and give up control in ways that benefit both the group and its individuals. The worker deals with confrontation in front of witnesses. The presence of witnesses carries a power in a culture where conflict is interpreted, convoluted, denied or smoothed over, mostly behind closed doors by the formal power holders.

When the group is worked by a practitioner with a grasp of the principles, the work of the group attains dimensions it cannot have otherwise (Kurland and Salmon, 2002). Purposeful application of group work skills and theory enables groups to move beyond the illusion of work where groups led by non-skilled facilitators often stall (Shulman, 1999). Effectual group workers make a "demand for work" (Schwartz, 1971, p. 11) and clients are guided to wholeheartedly work on the issues they came to work on with forthrightness and clarity.

Some of the factors that make a group a *social work group* are the awareness and employment of the following principles:

- *Inclusion and respect.* Groups validate every person's voice and honor each participant's view by exemplifying faith and belief in each individual's capability of constructive contributions (Kurland and Salmon, 2002; Dies, 1995).
- *Mutual aid.* Mutual aid involves fostering people's ability to conceptualize and to articulate their own needs, and to recognize and

respond to other group member's needs. The principle of mutual aid has been alluded to as the most important concept of group work (Northen and Kurland, 2001; Shulman, 1999; Steinberg, 2002). Mutual aid creates the conditions in which people can support and assist one another with their personal goals. Being able to recognize and empathize with others, to listen to others and express one's self, and see the commonalities with other group members empowers participants to interact more effectively in their varied social arenas (Schwartz, 1973; Shulman, 1999).

- *Stage Management.* Effective social group workers recognize and make use of the various stages of group development, and use the products and by products of energy generated by the interactions of the group in *beginnings*, *middles*, and *ends*. Studies show that group development can traverse these stages in a cyclical manner, and that timing interventions to stage development is important (Garvin, 2001; Shulman, 1999).

- *Use of Conflict.* Facing and exploring conflict is core to the expertise and effectiveness of group work (Bernstein, 1973; Northen and Kurland 2001). This can involve "tuning in" (Schwartz, 1971), or understanding euphemisms and codes that group members use, and helping members see contradictions, commonalities and differences.

- *Conscious development, use, and implications of purpose.* Skilled facilitators regularly bring members' awareness to defining and developing the group's changing purpose (Kurland and Salmon, 1997). Consistent agreement and crystallization of purpose adds to group cohesion and the group sense of self determination.

- *Breaking taboos.* Group work practitioners develop the ability to say the things people have the hardest time saying, and naming the "pink elephants" in the room. At times the things that some individuals regard as shameful, deviant, or abnormal are normalized by the practitioner's ability to break taboos (Shulman, 1999).

- *Value of activity.* Social learning theories have taught us that there are major differences in learning styles. Use of art, music, writing, playing, and acting are invaluable in reaching varied populations, meeting people where they are at, and using clients' strengths (Wright,1999; Northen and Kurland, 2001).

- *Problem-solving.* Practitioners regularly are called upon to guide the group through decision-making and problem-solving processes. A mistake commonly made by the non-educated group worker is to leap to resolution and solution of the presenting issue without benefiting group members with a proper exploration of the issue (Kurland and Salmon, 1999; Northen and Kurland, 2001), or framework to use in the future. Kurland and Salmon (1999) present a five-step process based on the work of John Dewey.

FORCES AT WORK

There are many factors that distinguish social group work from other groups. Social work groups are complex systems with multi-dimensional tasks. Group members assume different roles that generate varied interfacing and interactions. The effectual group creates norms and develops its own culture. An important tenet of social group work is that the group itself is an entity with its own lifecycle. Therefore the social group worker attends to each individual in the group as well as the group as a whole. There are dynamics, patterns, and stages evolving thru the life of a group, be it fifteen minutes, or fifteen months (Northen, 1987; Shulman, 1999; Garvin, 2001). Social workers' awareness of how people behave during each of those stages can greatly benefit any group. People are put at ease during *beginnings*, and encouraged to air conflict and explore issues to resolve problems during the *middle* stage by knowledgeable group work practitioners. Group workers learn to contextualize and point out contradictions, make connections, and illuminate bonds and differences advantageously.

A group worker can be working the group and creating the magic of groups without having a recognized leadership role. Staff meetings and meetings in general can become more effective groups as a result of a group worker being present using their skills (Rubin, 2002).

Dies (1995) found empirical evidence documenting the value of group work for clients suffering from alcoholism, sexual dysfunction, depression, schizophrenia, anxiety, and bereavement. Other populations that group work is used with include battered women, children, rape victims, victims of mass violence, people living with diseases, old people, and prisoners (Northen, 1987; Northen and Kurland, 2001). Types of groups that are utilized by social work practitioners include closed membership short or long-term groups, open short-term or long-term groups, support groups, psycho-therapy and activity groups.

EFFICACY

In a review of the literature addressing the effectiveness of group work, the pragmatic benefits mentioned included affordability to clients and staff efficiency (Dies, 1995; O'Conner, 2002). Dies (1995) cautions practitioners that the potential effects of group work may be watered down when agencies have waiting lists for individual services and offer groups as a second best alternative He further posits that the client's view of the treatment may impact its effectiveness and how agencies present the modality makes a difference. The likelihood of a group's success within an agency is compromised when the agency regards groups as non-essential. Unfortunately, agencies often cut groups first during uncertain financial times (Getzel, Kurland, and Salmon, 1986), sending a message that groups are adjunct to the work of the agency.

Groups foster an understanding that one is not alone in their suffering by universalizing the issues members face (Shaffer and Galinsky, 1989; Northen, 1987). Theorists recognize that the mutual sense of identification group members receive in groups fosters a sense of belonging (Northen, 1987; Shulman, 1999). Belonging and relating to a peer group reduces anxiety, increases self-expression and willingness to try new ideas (Northen, 1976; Shulman, 1999). Northen (1987) attributes an improvement in members' self-esteem to when they see that others who have the same problem are likeable.

A frequently mentioned benefit of mutual aid is the sense of altruism gained from helping others (Kaul and Badner, 1978; Steinberg, 2004). This includes the skills and abilities that group participants acquire to listen and understand others. Members learn to express helpful feedback, give support, share time responsibly, and explore differences and commonalities (Dies, 1995). Shaffer and Galinsky (1989) remark on the gains made when members can work through their relationships in the context of treatment, instead of just talking about them.

A reduction of problems is attributed to the validation members receive in groups as well as their opportunity to ventilate (Northen, 1987; Shulman, 1999). Theorists often allude to the fostering of hope that occurs in groups when members observe each other's progress, and the worker encourages members to share their coping strategies (Northen, 1992; Garvin, 1997). Members learn problem solving skills through employment of a consistent formula, and the successful resolution of conflict empowers them to deal with subsequent similar challenges (Bernstein, 1973; Northen and Kurland 2001).

Group work is empowering in its avoidance of patient-therapist dependency (Shaffer and Galinsky, 1989). The required power sharing that the worker must do in creating mutual aid groups strengthens the participant's sense of self-determination (Middleman, 1990; Gitterman and Shulman, 1994). A sense of ownership and investment in the group empowers participants.

THE CENTRALITY OF GROUP WORK IN SOCIAL WORK

Empowerment and strengths-based principles of the social work profession are fundamental in a perspective which conceptualizes the client's involvement as co-creators with the social worker (Falck, 1983). Empowerment is also conveyed by the message group work gives; that each individual has something constructive to contribute (Kurland and Salmon, 1996; Dies, 1995).

Schwartz (1971) defines social works' function as mediating the ". . . process thru which the individual and his society reach out to each other thru a mutual need for self-fulfillment." The overall goal for group participants is to become more effective in their lives within groups and systems to which they belong (Dies, 1995). These objectives place group work as foundational to the social work paradigm.

The work of social group work theorists and educators demonstrate why group work is an integral component of social work methodology. Social work with groups can be seen as an important step in a natural progression of social work services. This progression proceeds from casework to activism in the following manner:

Casework–Counseling–Group Work–Activism (Community Organizing)

Using Maslow's Hierarchy of Needs (1966) as a lens to conceptualize social work and its modalities, the mutual aid system of group work is an ideal medium in which to satisfy individuals' social needs for affection, belonging, acceptance, self-esteem, and actualization (Figure 1).

The idea of successful group work leading to action is not new. Greenfield and Rothman (1987) give several examples of groups that decided to stay together and become social networks for each other as well as political action groups. They suggest that "transformation" be added to the stages model of group, postulating that a defining a new

FIGURE 1. Maslow's Hierarchy of Needs.

Maslow's Hierarchy	Needs	Service	Method
Physical: Physiological Safety Protection	Food, housing, health care, legal intervention, crisis intervention, needs assessment (clinical, mental health, GAF*)	Referral and informationt Access to resources Casework Advocacy Counseling Screening	Casework Case management Counseling, Small group work Planning
Social: Affection Belonging Acceptance **Esteem:** Self respect Autonomy	Validation, support Feelings of belonging, acceptance, membership Feelings of hope, love, connectedness	Getting support from peers as well as the agency Breaking isolation Organizational involvement	Group Work (closed membership support groups, encourage intimate sharing and exploration, mutual aid); and/or open group work Activity groups
Self actualization: Doing Putting ideas into action	Resources, energy, connections, Friends, associates, social groups being with others	Political participation	Activity groups, community organizing macro groups, local, national, global Praxis (reflection plus action)

*GAF: Global Assessment of Functioning

purpose is highly plausible in a group that has experienced high cohesion, identification and strength (Greenfield and Rothman, 1987). In their view, the group itself progresses through Maslow's paradigm, and finds its self ready to act.

THE PROCESS OF REFLECTION

Part of the power of group work is in the reflection that occurs between each member of the group with each other and the group as a whole. The dynamic interchanges between each and all call forth the noticing of commonalities and differences, and a seeing of one's self in relationship. This multi-faceted mirror of perception between the individual and the group can create a powerful arena for creating self-awareness.

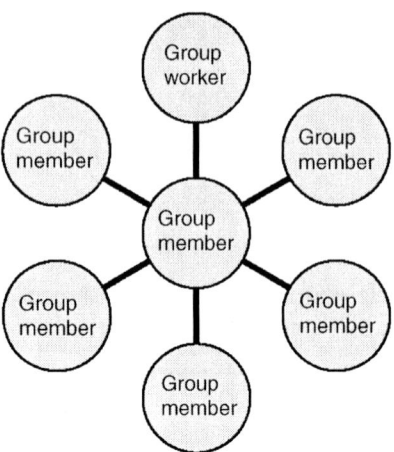

This portrayal of an individual's opportunity to view themselves in relation to other group members and the workers is replicated with each participant.

CASE EXAMPLE

The following case example illustrates the reflective process in a support group of lesbians between the ages of seventy and eighty-five. They have been meeting for two months and are struggling with issues of intimacy Wanting more meaningful friendships has been identified as an issue they want to struggle with. The group is an open one, meaning the membership configuration changes often, and new members may come and go.

At the group meeting prior, members shared memories of early rejection. Sheila, who is 74 years old, and a regular group member, has talked before in the group about feeling lonely. "I have to force myself to get up in the morning, because there is nothing for me to do," she has said to the group more than once. In this case example, Sheila initiates a continuation of last week's discussion:

> "I have been thinking a lot about rejection since the group last week. I remembered having two girlfriends when I was a child, and we always played together. One day I discovered them playing jacks without me, and having a good time. I never knew they

played without me. I felt so bad. I feel like people only want to be friends with me to a point. I think I am not creative or intellectual enough, I don't know, like something is missing. I know, I know, my self-esteem is horrible." Patricia replied by telling Sheila that now she understood better why Sheila hasn't responded to Patricia's efforts to reach out. "I thought you did not like me," Patricia said, "Now I get that it is your insecurity." Sheila was surprised. "Really? You really were trying to reach out to me?" When Patricia assured her she was, Sheila replied, "Well try again!" Jewelle, who has known Sheila for more than twenty years looks at Sheila with disbelief. "I can't believe what I am hearing! You are so bright and confident. I never would think you had a self-esteem problem!" At this point the worker pulls the rest of the group in by summarizing and reaching for full participation (Middleman (1990). "That is a great example of a misperception of how people see us! Has anyone else ever been misperceived, or think they misperceived someone, or some thing?" Jane answered. "I never know what people are thinking about me. I was never wanted as a child, I was told that a lot. I never talked about myself and I stifled my artistic expression, because I felt so bad about myself." The mutual aid process engages here, and Tania, a very brusque woman, who claims she does not want any friendships, tells Jane, "Now you can change that. You can let your creative self out now! You have us, you know." Patricia relates to Jane as well. "You know Jane, my mother hated me, too. I think I know what you went through. I hated myself for so long. I had to learn the mantra 'I am good, I am good, I am good,' and I still have to do that sometimes." Jane said, "I am glad I came today. I am glad someone understands."

Building on Patricia's offering, the worker asks the group if there were other things that group members do that help negative self-perceptions. Sheila remarked that talking about it helped her put it in perspective, but that, "It was a lot easier to tell stories like that when we were younger." Jane agreed. "I think we keep the painful stuff in, and the more time goes by, the more we keep things in, until we hardly speak at all anymore." At this point, Rita, who has said nothing until now, tells about a childhood of severe and prolonged abuse, and then an abusive sexual relationship. "Now I watch people a long time before I get close to them. I want to see how they treat others first. I never talk about this stuff, you are right, Jane. We keep it stuffed." The worker commended the insight and the risk taking of the group members and asked Jane if there was anything more she wanted to share with the group. Jane said there wasn't, and then goes on to say, "But I am very depressed you know. My mother always told me she wished she aborted me. She was very mean." At this revelation, Tania explodes, "Your mother was a bitch! She had no right to be so fucking mean to you!" Jane smiled for the first time in weeks and said, "No she didn't, did she?"

In this short example of a group interaction, the mutual aid process is evident in the support and validation members are giving each other. Group members reflect their impressions and observations as well as their own related experiences to their peers. Sheila received input on how she is seen by others, Tania breaks through her detachment to support Jane, and Patricia and Rita share painful experiences that have created obstacles to intimacy in their lives. The fullness of the empathetic understanding these women experienced in this group could not be matched in individual sessions.

CONCLUSION

Contemporary society's social workers face a vast array of challenges posed by the marginalization, isolation, deprivation, and stereotyping of the populations we work with. Social group work methodology and its principles exert extraordinary effectiveness in contradicting feelings of powerlessness and internalized self-hatred, and improving social functioning. It is alarming that this valuable social work method faces the danger of being diffused and robbed of its potency, of its magic when we need it most.

Group work is grounded in a substantial theoretical framework that has been established over the course of the last century. It is the embodiment of social work ethics and principles in action. The fact that the theory and skill base of methodology is in danger of becoming extinct in practice and social work education should create an outrage among all social work professionals. CSWE and NASW must be held accountable and pressured to ensure adequate group work theory and methodology is included in social work curricula.

Educational resources for those who wish to specialize in group work need to be established within schools of social work. The needs of people who are facilitating groups without education and training must be considered. Continuing education courses in group work are needed for para-professionals as well as for Masters of Social Work who did not receive adequate instruction. San Diego State University, in conjunction with AASWG (2003) has created a model of this type of training.

It is apparent that groups have generative power when one considers the multi-dimensional, multiplying potentiality of social group work. This paper only touched upon the most basic reasons for group work to be used for individual change work. There is an equally compelling case for the role of group work in social change that has been made by leading educators and practitioners in the field (Gitterman, 2003; Getzel, 2003; Henry, 2003). When viewing the possibilities, the imagination can conceive of an exponential capacity for global understanding and change through the medium of social work groups.

There is an alarming trend in the devolution of group work as an effective and viable modality in the field of social work as evidenced by its invisibility in most of the social work foundational curricula and direct practice. Kurland and Salmon's (1992, 1996, 2002, 2004) warning that group work theory and principles may be absorbed into the generalist practice is one not to be reflected upon lightly. Rather it must be a catalyst for those of us who believe passionately in the magic and the power of group work to create a movement that elevates the method to its rightful central place before the practice of true social group work reaches its extinction.

REFERENCES

Bernstein, S. (1973). Conflict and group work. *Explorations in group work.* Boston: Charles River Books, pp. 72-106.

Birnbaum, M.L. and Auerbach, C. (1994). Group work in graduate social work education: The price of neglect. *Journal of Social Work Education*, 36 (2): 347-356.

Cohen, C.S. (1995). Making it happen: From great idea to successful support group. *Social Work with Groups*, 18 (1): 67-80.

Cohen, M.B. and Mullender, A. (1999). The personal in the political: Exploring the group work continuum from individual to social change goals. *Social Work with Groups*, 22 (1): 18-31.

Dies, R. R. (1995). Group psychotherapies. In Gurman, A., and Messer, S. *Essential psychotherapies: Theory and practice.* New York: The Guilford Press, pp. 515-550.

Flexner, A. (1915) Is social work a profession? In *Proceedings of the National Conference of Charities and Corrections* (pp. 576-590). Chicago: National Conference on Charities and Correction.

Garvin, C. (2001). The potential impact of small-group research on social group work practice. In Kelly, T., Berman-Rossi, T., Palombo, S. (Eds.). *Group work: Strategies for strengthening resiliency.* New York: The Haworth Press, Inc., pp. 51-70.

Getzel, G. (2003). Group work and social justice: Rhetoric or action? In Sullivan, N., Mesbur, E. S., Lang, N., Goodman, G., Mitchell, L. (Eds). *Social work with groups: Social justice through personal, community and societal change.* New York: The Haworth Press, Inc., pp. 53-64.

Getzel, G., Kurland, R., and Salmon, R. (1987). Teaching and learning the practice of social group work: Four curriculum tools. In J. Lassner, K. Powell, Finnegan, E. (Eds.). *Social group work: Competence and values in practice.* New York: The Haworth Press, Inc., pp. 35-49.

Gitterman, A. (2003). The meaning, scope, and context of the concept of social justice in social work with groups. In Sullivan, N., Mesbur, E. S., Lang, N., Goodman, G., Mitchell, L. (Eds). *Social work with groups: Social justice through personal, community and societal change.* New York: The Haworth Press, Inc., pp. 25-34.

Greenfield, W., and Rothman, B. (1987). Termination or transformation? Evolving beyond termination in groups. In J. Lassner, K. Powell, Finnegan, E. (Eds.). *Social group work: Competence and values in practice.* New York: The Haworth Press, Inc., pp. 51-66.

Henry, S. (2003). Social group work, social justice. In Sullivan, N., Mesbur, E. S., Lang, N., Goodman, G., Mitchell, L. (Eds). *Social work with groups: Social justice through personal, community and societal change.* New York: The Haworth Press, Inc., pp. 65-78.

Kurland, R., and Salmon, R. (1992). Group work vs. casework in a group: Principles and implications for teaching and practice. *Social Work with Groups,* 15 (4): 3-14.

Kurland, R., and Salmon, R. (1998). Purpose: A misunderstood and misused keystone of group work practice. *Social Work with Groups,* 21 (3): 5-17.

Kurland, R., and Salmon, R. (1992). Making a joyful noise: Presenting, promoting and portraying group work to and for the profession. *Plenary presentation at the 14th annual symposium of the association for the advancement of social work with groups.* Atlanta, Georgia. Also in (1996) Stempler, B., Glass, M. (Eds.) *Social group work today and tomorrow: Moving from theory to advanced training and practice.* New York: The Haworth Press, Inc. pp. 19-32.

Kurland, R., and Salmon, R. (2002). Caught in the doorway between education and practice: group work's battle for survival. *Plenary presentation at the 24th annual symposium of the association for the advancement of social work with groups.* Brooklyn, New York. Also In Press, Cohen, C., Philips, M., and Hanson, M. (Eds.) *Think group: Strength and diversity in group work.* New York: The Haworth Press, Inc.

Kurland, R., and Salmon, R. (1999). *Teaching a methods course in social work with groups.* Alexandria, VA: The Council on Social Work Education, Inc.

Kurland R., and Salmon R., (2004). The survival of social group work: A call to action. *Social Work with Groups,* 27 (1): 3-16.

Magen, R. (1998). Practice with groups. In Mattiani, M., Lowry, C., Meyer, C. (Eds.). *The foundations of social work practice.* Washington, DC: NASW Press, pp. 108-208.

Middleman, R. (1980). The use of program: Review and update. *Social Work with Groups,* 3 (3): 5-23.

Middleman, R. and Wood, G. G. (1990). *Skills for direct practice in social work.* New York: Columbia University Press.

Middleman, R.R. (1990, October). Group work and the heimlich maneuver: Unchoking social work education. In Fike, D., and Rittner, B. (Eds.). *Working from strengths: The essence of group work.* Miami Shores: Center for Group Work Studies, pp. 16-40.

Northen, H. and Kurland, R. (2001) *Social work with groups.* (3rd ed.) New York: Columbia University Press.

Northen, H. (1976). Psychosocial Practice in Small Groups. In Roberts, R. and Northen, H. *Theories of social work with groups,* NY: Columbia University Press.

Northen, H. (1987). Selection of groups as the preferred modality of practice. In J. Lassner, K. Powell, and Finnegan, E. (Eds.). *Social group work: Competence and values in practice.* New York: The Haworth Press, Inc., pp. 19-34.

O'Conner, D. L. (2002). Toward empowerment: Re-visioning family support groups. *Social Work with Groups,* 25 (4): 37-46.

Rubin, M. (2002). Making curriculum purposeful in group work with persons with severe mental illnesses. In S. Henry, J. East, and C. Schmitz (Eds.). *Social work with groups: Mining the gold.* (2002) New York: The Haworth Press, Inc., pp. 163-183.

San Diego State University and AASWG (2003). *Maximizing outcomes by mastering group work skills.* 224 Hannalei Drive, Vista, CA.

Schwartz, W. (1971). On the use of groups in social work practice. In W. Schwartz and Z.R. Zalba (Eds.). *The practice of group work.* New York: Columbia University Press, pp. 3-24.

Shaffer and Galinsky, M. (1989) *Models of group therapy* (2nd ed). Engelwood Cliffs, NJ: Prentice Hall.

Shulman, L. (1999). *The skills of helping individuals, families, groups and communities.* (4th ed.) Itsaca, IL: F.E.Peacock Publishers, Inc.

Steinberg, D.M. (1993). Some findings from a study on the impact of group work education on social practitioners' work with groups. *Social Work with Groups,* 16 (3): 23-39.

Steinberg, D. M. (2002). The magic of mutual aid. *Social Work with Groups.* 25 (1/2): 31-39.

Steinberg, D. M. (2004). *The mutual aid approach to working with groups: Helping people help one another.* (2nd. ed.) New York: The Haworth Press, Inc.

Wright, W. (1999). The use of purpose in on-going activity groups: A framework for maximizing the therapeutic impact. *Social Work with Groups,* 22 (2/3): 31-54.

The Art, Science, Heart, and Ethics of Social Group Work: Lessons from a Great Teacher

Dominique Moyse Steinberg

SUMMARY. This article highlights the components of Professor Roselle Kurland's vision that she made contagious to all who would listen. She believed that good group work requires a blend of science and art. In addition, she advocated for "heart" in practice and without exception held social workers accountable to the highest possible standards of both human and professional ethics. She believed that human ethics were central and essential to professional ethics. *[Article copies available for a fee from The Haworth Document Delivery Service: 1-800-HAWORTH. E-mail address: <docdelivery@haworthpress.com> Website: <http://www.Haworth Press.com> © 2006 by The Haworth Press, Inc. All rights reserved.]*

KEYWORDS. Group work, ethics, social work education, Roselle Kurland, art and science

INTRODUCTION

In spring of 2005 Roselle Kurland, one of the great teachers of all time, passed away–an untimely and unexpected loss, and a loss that will affect the whole of the social work profession, not just the world of so-

[Haworth co-indexing entry note]: "The Art, Science, Heart, and Ethics of Social Group Work: Lessons from a Great Teacher." Steinberg, Dominique Moyse. Co-published simultaneously in *Social Work with Groups* (The Haworth Press, Inc.) Vol. 29, No. 2/3, 2006, pp. 33-45; and: *Making Joyful Noise: The Art, Science, and Soul of Group Work* (ed: Andrew Malekoff, Robert Salmon, and Dominique Moyse Steinberg) The Haworth Press, Inc., 2006, pp. 33-45. Single or multiple copies of this article are available for a fee from The Haworth Document Delivery Service [1-800-HAWORTH, 9:00 a.m. - 5:00 p.m. (EST). E-mail address: docdelivery@haworthpress.com].

cial group work. Teacher of group work (along with research methods and professional writing) at Hunter College School of Social Work in New York City, Roselle Kurland traveled around the United States and Canada for over 20 years, helping social workers to understand the power and beauty of groups, to develop and refine their skill level in working with groups, and to deepen their appreciation for the ways in which group work translates the fundamental mandates of social work into action: the mandate for a holistic perspective, by recognizing the total person in each group member; the mandate for a strength-centered practice base, by using group process to constantly promote mutual aid; and the mandate to respect self determination, by insisting that relevance and nothing but relevance dictate the purpose and course of any group.

In short, Roselle Kurland created a legacy unsurpassed and one, like those of all master teachers, that has both vertical and horizontal ripple effects. Vertical ripples carry forward to future generations of social workers through her written work, and through her students and their students the art, science, heart, and ethics of group work practice as she saw it. Horizontal ripples carried in her lifetime a legacy to all who came into contact with her long enough to catch her vision and become contagious with her brand of group work. Her untimely death leaves a multitude of social workers–even legions, it might be said–to cry out in their respective worlds of work on her behalf and that of her long-time friend and collaborator Robert Salmon (and to mix their metaphors): "Into the Breach Once Again, Dear Friends. Let's Make Joyful Noise! (1996). Let's promote social group work!" And to that end, this paper attempts to highlight the special legacy of Roselle Kurland and to capture its essence: the theories, concepts, and principles of group work practice that she embodied and promoted with every instructional breath and that her students carry forth on her behalf.

What *was* social group work to Roselle Kurland? First, she believed that good group work requires a blend of science and art. In addition, she advocated for "heart" in practice and without exception held social workers accountable to the highest possible standards of both human and professional ethics. I include "human" here as well as "professional," because to Roselle Kurland human ethics were central and essential to professional ethics.

One example of this professional ideology of ethics is reflected in one of her earliest cautions to students around the immorality of hidden agendas, those service or treatment agendas that practitioners develop but do not share explicitly with group members–agendas on the sly, as it were, unspoken plans for others. "If you can't say it to someone, you have no right to do it," students would hear her say year after year as they struggled with the discomfort of acknowledging in explicit ways some of the more sensitive topics they encountered in their social work practice, as they struggled with speaking about the normally unspeakable or with giving light to taboo subjects, subjects that are often the very raisons d'etre of group work.

I first heard this when I wrote in my very first class log assignment, "I worry about making some things explicit. I was brought up to be polite–to be sensitive, and I'm afraid I will embarrass them if I point out a problem." Her response was loud and clear. If I could not acknowledge in words the reason that people need my services then of course I couldn't help them. That simple response struck me like a thunderbolt. "If you can't say it you have no right to do it"–a lifetime lesson in professional AND human ethics. If our groups remain "polite," she said, then they would be no different from many of the other groups to which people belong–no more real, no more respectful, no more useful.

With certitude, then, the students of Roselle Kurland know that it takes four ingredients: skill, art, heart, and ethical sensitivity–to carry out good group work. Contrary to popular belief and perhaps even in juxtaposition to the politically correct tendency to insist on the unconsidered equality of all things, there are NOT several approaches to group work all of them equally good; there is good group work, and there are bad habits!

Actually, Roselle Kurland's legacy is obviously and clearly identified in another paper–her last paper delivered at the 26th Symposium of the Association for the Advancement of Social Work With Groups in Detroit, Michigan–in which she identified what she believed to be the keys to "superb practice." She giggled with absolute delight when she told me that she was using the word "superb" to describe what can happen to already good practice if group workers would pay special attention to a few key aspects of practice, such as planning and group purpose, stage theory, group work vs. casework in a group (1992), effective problem solving, and the changing role of the practitioner over a group's lifetime.

Organized around the art, science, heart, and ethics of social work with groups, this paper now takes that last paper a step further by highlighting those components of her vision that I believe she made contagious to all who would listen, or otherwise said, what her students know.

THE ART OF GROUP WORK

What do Roselle Kurland's students know about the "art" of group work? First, we know that practice *is* artful. Artful practice seeks to understand the relationship between context and possibility–to dance the perpetual dance between what is and what might be. It knows about "tuning in." Artful practice knows how to make group work take shape in any environment, how to make it appealing in even hostile settings. That is the art of practice in a broad sense. On a smaller scale artful practice touches many areas of work. It reads between the lines. For example, it listens with a keen ear to people's desires as well as needs and blends both into developing group purpose. It pays attention to people's complexities–their desire for individuality *and* belonging, for taking *and* contributing, for commonality *and* difference, for structure *and* space, for safety *and* creativity. Artful group work practice is a keen observer, sensitive to the possibility of change–to nuances in group climate that herald a change in needs and desires over time–and thus, artful group work is open to change. In fact, truly artful practice even anticipates changes in climate so that changes can be made proactively rather than reactively or belatedly, or as is too often the case, belligerently, or not at all.

Artful group workers are brilliant mathematicians, so brilliant that they can sum two plus two into five, an empirically impossible but spiritually accurate calculation that happens every time strangers are helped to develop into a community with strength and potential that is exponentially greater than the sum of its individual members. It might be argued by some that this impossible task belongs to scientific practice rather than artful practice, but science and art have long been kindred spirits, and so perhaps it can be said that scientific practice discovered the equation and that artful practice knows how to make it come true!

Artful group work is also in style and in smile, in attention to the sense of things, in the vision of a problem reframed as opportunity, in the manner of conveying faith in people's ability to positively affect their lives. An artfully developed contract speaks to what its participants might, can, and should do for one another rather than what they should not do. In sum, artful practice is a large part of the "Kurland approach" to group work practice: the small ways in which we attempt to engage people, the verbal and nonverbal ways in which we show we care–the touch, the handshake, the ways in which we express faith–the nod of understanding, the many ways in which we use ourselves as barometers to help others and to understand others–the wrinkle of a brow to show we are listening and concentrating, and the ways in which we show respect for effort. It is the ability to communicate verbally and nonverbally our love and respect for this method of helping we call group work and for those it touches. Artful practice is the elegant part of social work with groups.

THE SCIENCE OF GROUP WORK

Students of Roselle Kurland also know that there is science to group work, that scientific group work is based on amalgamating many areas of knowledge including individual physical, sexual, cognitive, and moral development and behavior; social, political, and economic dynamics, norms, mores, and behavior that dictate and change our understanding of social work; the nature and function of systems large and small; group development theories; theories that propose frameworks for understanding our intrapsychic structures; theories that guide self help, interaction, and mutual aid; theories that categorize personality types; theories of self image and theories of social image; culturally-based theories, racially-oriented theories, gender-specific theories, old-age-related theories; individual growth and change theories; social force theories; leadership models; and decision-making models–to identify but some of the growing body of knowledge on which good group work rests. Scientific group work is eclectic, taking from all of these theories and more that which can help to shape group process into one that takes from and gives to each group member the best there is, however defined–that catalyzes mutual aid.

Consider group development. Years of giving on-site workshops to social work agencies confirm that the several theories of group progression are relatively unknown and yet, knowledge that all groups develop over time, regardless of which particular theoretical lens is used to understand that progression, is considered essential to good practice. In fact, I have heard stage theory referred to as the group worker's bible! Stage tells us where group members "are" at any given moment in their physical, emotional, and spiritual relationships to one another, to the group, to the worker, and to their overall environment; it tells us what needs to happen as a result of where they "are" in order to help the group move from group (collectivity) to Group (community); and it tells us what we need to do in order to make whatever needs to happen, happen.

Scientific group work also draws on a variety of models for practice so that approach to practice can be professional rather than technocratic, so that we do not reinvent the wheel every single time we encounter a new group. Using a planning model, for instance, helps us to set the stage for group relevance and success. In fact, Roselle Kurland's well known model (1978), which she developed as her doctoral dissertation, is one of her major contributions to the profession.

Other models contribute to good practice as well. Strength-centered problem-solving models (Kurland and Salmon, 1992; Somers, 1976), for example, help us to carry out the professional mandate of finding and building on whatever people have to offer on their own behalf. Psychosocial models of practice (Breton, 1994, 1995; Newstetter, 1935; Northen and Kurland, 2001; Steinberg, 2004; Wilson and Ryland, 1949) help to insure that we invite whole persons to participate in, and their whole life experiences to contribute to, our groups. Models for intervening in group process help to prevent us from carrying out aggregational therapy of individuals (Berman-Rossi, 1993; Hartford, 1971; Northen and Kurland, 2001; Steinberg, 1996). Models for instilling democracy in our groups help insure that the many principles of social work practice, such as informed consent and self determination are translated from ideals to real-world action (Bernstein, 1973; Galinsky and Schopler, 1977; Glassman and Kates, 1990; Konopka, 1978).

Additionally, an ever growing body of group-specific skills help scientific practice include knowledge of the ideal, helps to lend structure to why we say and do what we say and do in our work with groups, and helps us to evaluate just how close our reality is to the ideal (Henry, 1992; Middleman and Wood, 1990; Phillips, 1957; Robinson, 1942; Steinberg, 2004). We know that group work skills range from the formal, such as assessment of the environment and making deliberate composition choices, to the informal, such as "hanging out" and "shmoozing." Yes, every single student of Roselle Kurland knows that "hanging out" and "shmoozing" are, in fact, distinct and valid group- specific skills!

Finally, the many concepts contained in the theories upon which we draw, such as inclusion and membership (Bernstein, 1976; Falck, 1988), leadership (Trecker, 1955; Schwartz and Zalba, 1971), tuning in (Shulman, 1999), dual focus (Shulman, 1999; Steinberg, 2004), purpose (Kurland and Salmon, 1998; Northen and Kurland, 2001), relevance (Schwartz and Zalba, 1971), relationship (Coyle, 1949, 1959) authority (Glassman and Kates, 1983; Kurland and Salmon, 1993), contribution (Breton, 1989), contract (Northen and Kurland, 2004), goals and norms (Galinsky and Schopler, 1971; Roman, 2002; Steinberg, 2004), consensus (Glassman and Kates, 1990), and nonverbal communication (Middleman, 1982) guide our approach to practice regardless of population, purpose, or setting. We know, for example, that group purpose–or the *why* of any group–is what keeps vision in sight and prevents a group from simply being a chain of encounters where people may enjoy themselves but after which they cannot really articulate the point of it.

In short, scientific group work is based on a broad body of knowledge that lifts practice above common everyday wisdom or intuition into purposeful action, that helps initial reaction change to deliberate response, that transforms practice from potentially technocratic tedium to theoretically defensible skill. It draws on the ever evolving literature on group work. It contributes to the ever evolving literature on group work. It is reflected in all words and deeds that are anchored in information, and it is reflected in the informed decisions we make about the kinds of groups we develop and the nature of the vision we offer them.

Finally, scientific group work insists on reaching for ideals in spite of a constantly compromising reality and on finding ways to apply those ideals, even if we do so with modulation. For example, although planning is often neglected in the fast-paced world of today, once the science of it is known, the practitioner has an ideal against which the real can be measured, against which questions can be asked, and even against which the consequences of having a lack of opportunity to plan can be weighed. It is not because teachers love to torture that the famous "Records of Service" are assigned to unhappy group work students year after year in order to help them critique their skills! It is precisely because there is a science to group work, a science that can be discovered, passed on, and learned. Scientific practice is the knowledge-based part of social work with groups.

THE HEART OF GROUP WORK

In addition to art and science, good group work includes "heart." What does it mean to practice group work with "heart?" Heartfelt group work begins and ends with faith in the capacity of people to contribute to the quality of their own destinies. "Have faith in the group!"–one of Roselle Kurland's most frequent rallies, epitomizes this important aspect of social group work. Heartfelt group work believes in people, in potential, in effort, in the value and reward of contribution, in the search for common ground, in the wealth that is diversity, in the power of "we-ness," of community. Heartfelt group work even believes in magic (Steinberg, 2002).

Heartfelt group work recognizes the complexities of individuals and vagaries of social life. It pays close attention to subtlety, to nuance, to the "edges" of things, to human fears, fancies, and frailties. It takes in and integrates into approach to practice the full context of life, the feeling states of both our inner and outer environments. It "gets" that we are both excited and ambivalent in new experiences. It can tell when we have the jitters and knows how to deal with them. It understands nervous banter and knows how to put us at ease. Heartfelt group work loves to set the stage, to set up the scene, and to move into the shadows once the play begins and the actors learn their lines.

Heartfelt group work is never afraid of other people's strength. It is happy to lead sometimes and at other times, to share the reins. It is confident, never jealous, and applauds–purposefully, loudly, and unabashedly–when a group takes charge of its affairs or navigates choppy waters on its own. Heartfelt group work has *faith*!

Heartfelt group work is not afraid of honesty, nor does it impose hidden agendas. It welcomes the kinds of conversations that most of us cannot have in our every day lives, and it believes, truly believes, that good group experiences–experiences that include clarity, consensus, and purpose–can enrich our lives beyond measure. It *knows* it!

Heartfelt group work is empathic. It understands that people cannot engage in self reflection much less entertain new possibilities in an atmosphere of judgment. It knows that people always learn, grow, and change more successfully and with greater commitment, ownership, and long-lasting effects if they do so in a climate of support, not criticism (Konopka, 1983). When confrontation is necessary, therefore, heartfelt group work always confronts with the desire to help, not to deride and with empathy–with, as Northen and Kurland (2001) put it, "an arm around the shoulder."

Heartfelt group work enjoys discovery, expression, and enjoyment; it encourages the imagination to run wild and people to find meaning in ways that may well be different from ours. It does not seek constant sameness. Thus, it constantly promotes what Glassman and Kates (1990) call a "democratic-humanistic" group climate, a climate in which many voices can be heard and where decisions come from those who will be most touched by them.

Finally, heartfelt group work loves the practitioner as well as the practice. It accepts the practitioner as just another human being in the mix, not as inherently better or obviously more "right" or "moral" or more "expert" or as "be-all/end-all" of group success. In its charity, heartfelt group work relieves the practitioner from carrying alone the burden for group success. It says, "We are in it together. I bring something. You bring something. Together, we can make good things happen." In short, heartfelt group work believes wholeheartedly in the value of we-ness–of groupness; and it *feels* for everyone's humanity, including the worker's. Finally, heartfelt group work believes that whatever needs to be done, it can surely be done *better* in groups!

Although Kurland and Salmon (1999) identify different types of learners, I believe that this particular aspect of practice is innate. One either buys into the proposition that we are all really "in it together" and "there but for fortune go I" or one does not. Those who do will have no difficulty incorporating heart into practice, translating with ease and comfort the values in reaching for other people's strengths, in inviting whole persons to participate in the group, and in developing relationships that have some take for the practitioner as well as give. Heartfelt practice knows that when the fundamental values of social work are realized, the magic of mutual aid can happen. Heartfelt practice is the magical part of social work with groups.

THE ETHICS OF GROUP WORK

Finally, we come to ethical group work practice–the belief in people's right to decide things for themselves, to be informed consumers of what our particular service industry offers, and the translation at every opportunity of that belief into action. Roselle Kurland's students know that it is only in a climate of good will and open information that people can make meaningful decisions. Should they join the group we have in mind? It depends. They need an honest tally of perspectives and expectations: theirs, ours, and those of the system in which the group is to operate in order to make an informed decision. Should they stay in a group? It depends. They have the right to assess the relevance of purpose, process, and content and the nature of common ground with the other members. Should they entertain new ways of being or doing or thinking? It depends. They have the right to examine problems and possibilities in a climate of good will, a climate that may include criticism but does not include punishment.

Ethical group work knows that people have the right to shape their own destinies, that the role of the social worker is to create space for that to happen, not to impose some traditionally or systematically or culturally sanctioned idea of how people's lives should look. Ethical group work demands the practitioner's *relevance*, whether it be biological, psychological, social, cultural, or spiritual. It also recognizes that the reason we provide structure is to help the contributions, creativity, and spontaneity of others to take place, not to prevent them from taking place. Roselle's statement, "If you can't say it, you do not have the right to do it" is a statement about ethical practice, that practice is not something that ever gets done *to* people but with and for people. That's why ethical group work seeks to work with groups rather than to lead them or worse yet to run them or worst of all, to *do* them! Does one *do* individuals, asks ethical group work? Hopefully not! Then why should we *do* groups??

Ethical group work understands that the purpose of any and every professional encounter should be both conceptualized and assessed from the point of view of all participants and their significant others. It pays keen attention to the environment and comes to arms when advocacy is needed. Ethical group work mediates between individuals and systems, but it is never a neutral participant. It is always biased, biased in favor of quality. It accepts as inevitable that authoritarian organizations parade as social service agencies, but it does not accept authoritarian practice. Instead, it encourages shared authority over group affairs and promotes group-based skills and strengths for decision making and problem solving. It promotes autonomy to the best of people's capacity in every group, the well and not so well, the adult and no so adult, the able and not so able, and takes to heart Virginia Robinson's admonition to treat the material at hand with greatest respect and sensitivity (1942).

Ethical group work understands that group purpose always belongs to the group, that there are consequences to imposing purpose. It knows that group purpose is a changing thing, that it cannot ever be written in stone. It may entertain curriculum-based practice, but it rails against curriculum-driven practice.

Ethical group work recognizes that risk taking, rehearsal, and learning are processes, not statuses, and that they can only emerge in a climate of mutuality and respect for effort. It encourages participation through example, not force. It does not reserve the right to say, "Do as I preach," but instead, in one way or another, models whatever it asks of group members.

Finally, ethical group work believes in informed consumerism and promotes accountability: the practitioner's accountability to the group as well as to the profession and group members' accountability to one another. It notices all bad habits–both personal and institutional–and fights for change through training, advocacy, or other form of social action. It fights for logic between expectations of practice and the lifeline of a group and fights against all mandates that either set us up to fail or that insist on simplistic practice.

The world of ethics and standards is one area in which the students of Roselle Kurland know that she was *not* generous. As teacher and mentor Roselle Kurland was generous without limit, but when it came to professional standards, she was rigid, relentless, and uncompromising–not generous. In group work practice she completely coveted the art of it, the science of it, the heart of it, and the ethic of it. In no one area was she willing to relent, give in, or even just slip a little. There was a bar, and that bar did not move. One was either above it or below it. And to those who slipped below she was uncharitable. This does not mean that she did not understand the incessant and inevitable tug of war between the ideal and the real. It means that her idea of good group work practice was to help the real strive for the ideal, not to just resign to the real without a fight. That the bar was rigid also does not mean that she did not understand and accept the struggles and mistakes inherent in any learning process. As long as her students gave it their best, she was very accepting. One of her favorite lines was that group work is so complex she did not ever expect her students to stop making mistakes, she just wanted their mistakes to become increasingly more sophisticated!

Thus, the students of Roselle Kurland know that professional practice means to strive for the ideal even when the real world impinges, which of course it always does in some way or other. They ask when and how to mediate, not if. They ask when and how to advocate, not if. They ask when and how to fight for change, not if. Ethical practice is the humane part of social work with groups.

CONCLUSION

In the end, the students of Roselle Kurland know that to be a good group worker is to be a juggler: to juggle art, science, heart, and ethics, so that they all come into play at once, for they are all needed at once. None of these alone is enough to make for good group work. We all know that good will is not enough to be a good group worker, but as Helen Phillips (1954) said, neither is skill alone enough. One can be ethical and still not know group work. On the other hand, one can know the science of group work–its skill and techniques–and like the pianist who plays with technical brilliance but without soul, still not be able to create the kinds of groups that people want to join. Roselle Kurland believed that it takes all of these ingredients to make good group work: knowledge and skill, yes, which can be learned, yes, but also humility, heart, and passion, all of which she unflinchingly and relentlessly attempted year after year, and each year with renewed hope and enthusiasm, to pass on to her students. This, we know.

REFERENCES

Berman-Rossi, T. (1993). The tasks and skills of the social worker across stages of group development, *Social Work with Groups*, 15(1-2), 69-81.

Bernstein, S. (1976). Values and group work, in S. Bernstein, ed., *Explorations in group work*, 72-106. Boston, MA: Boston University School of Social Work.

Bernstein, S. (1993). What happened to self-determination? *Social Work with Groups*, 16(1-2), 3-15.

Breton, M. (1989). Liberation theology, group work, and the right of the poor and oppressed to participate in the life of the community. *Social Work with Groups*, 12(3), 5-17.

Breton, M. (1994). On the meaning of empowerment and empowerment-oriented social work practice, *Social Work with Groups*, 17(3), 23-37.

Breton, M. (1995). The potential for social action in groups, *Social Work with Groups*, 18(2-3), 5-14.

Coyle, G. (1949). Definition of the function of the group worker. *The Group*, 11(3), 11-13.

Coyle, G. (1959). Some basic assumptions about group work, in M. Murphy, ed., *Curriculum study*, 11, 88-105. New York: Council on Social Work Education.

Falck, H. (1988). The management of membership: Social group work contributions, *Social Work with Groups*, 12(3), 19-32.

Galinsky, M. and Schopler, J. (1971). The practice of group goal formulation in social work practice. *Social Work Practice*, 24-32.

Galinsky, M. and Schopler, J. (1977). Warning: Groups may be dangerous. Social Work, 22(2), 89-94.

Glassman, U. and Kates, L. (1983). Authority themes and worker-group transactions: additional dimensions to the stages of group development. *Social Work with Groups*, 6(2), 33-52.

Glassman, U. and Kates, L. (1990). *Group work: A humanistic approach*. Newbury Park: Sage Publications.

Hartford, M. (1971). *Groups in social work*. New York: Columbia University Press.

Henry, S. (1992). *Group skills in social work: A four-dimensional approach*, 2nd ed. Pacific Grove, CA: Brooks/Cole Publishing Company.

Konopka, G. (1983). *Social group work: A helping process*, 3rd ed. Englewood Cliffs, NJ: Prentice Hall.

Kurland, R. (1978). Planning: The neglected component of group development, *Social Work with Groups*, 1(2), 173-178.

Kurland, R. and Salmon, R. (1999). Education for the group worker's reality: The special qualities and world view of those drawn to work with groups. *Journal of Teaching in Social Work*, 19(1-2), 123-137.

Kurland, R. and Salmon, R. (1992). Group work vs. casework in a group: Principles and implications for teaching and practice. *Social Work with Groups*, 15(4), 3-14.

Kurland, R. and Salmon, R. (1996). Making joyful noise: Presenting, promoting, and portraying group work to and for the profession, in B. Stempler and M. Glass, eds., *Social group work today and tomorrow: Moving from theory to advanced training and practice*, 19-32. Binghamton, NY: The Haworth Press, Inc.

Kurland, R. and Salmon, R. (1993). Not just one of the gang: Group workers and their role as an authority, in S. Wenocur et. al., eds., *Social work with groups: Expanding horizons*. Binghamton, NY: The Haworth Press, Inc.

Kurland, R. and Salmon, R. (1998). Purpose: A misunderstood and misused keystone of group work practice, *Social Work with Groups*, 21(3), 5-17.

Middleman, R. (1982). *The non-verbal method in working with groups*. Hebron, CT: Practitioner's Press.

Middleman, R. and Wood, G. G. (1990). *Skills for direct practice in social work*. New York: Columbia University Press.

Newstetter, W. (1935). What is social group work? *Proceedings of the national conference of social work*, 291-299.

Northen, H. and Kurland, R. (2001). *Social work with groups*, 3rd ed. New York: Columbia University Press.

Phillips, H. (1957). *Essentials of social group work skill*. New York: Association Press.

Robinson, V. (1942). *Training for skill in social casework*. Philadelphia, PA: University of Pennsylvania Press.

Roman, C. (2002). It is not always easy to sit on your mouth. *Social Work with Groups*, 25(1-2), 61-64.

Schwartz, W. and Zalba, Z. (1971). *The practice of group work*. New York: Columbia University Press.

Shulman, L. (1999). *The skills of helping individuals, families, groups, and communities*, 4th ed., Itasca, IL.: F. E. Peacock Publishers, Inc.

Somers, M. L. (1976). Problem-solving in small groups, in eds. R. Roberts and H. Northen, *Theories of social work with groups*, 331-367. New York: Columbia University Press.

Steinberg, D. M. (2002). The magic of mutual aid. *Social Work with Groups*, 25(1-2), 31-38.

Steinberg, D. M. (2004). *The mutual-aid approach to working with groups: Helping people help one another*, 2nd ed. Binghamton, NY: The Haworth Press, Inc.

Steinberg, D. M. (1996). She's doing all the talking, so what's in it for me? The use of time in mutual-aid groups, *Social Work with Groups*, 19(2), 5-16.

Trecker, H. (1955). *Group work: Foundations and frontiers*. New York: Whiteside, Inc.

Wilson, G. and Ryland, G. (1949). *Social group work practice*. Boston, MA: Houghton Mifflin and Company.

On Being Bold, Valuing Process, and Cultivating Collegiality

Keren Ludwig

Priska Imberti

SUMMARY. Professor Roselle Kurland's use of self was exemplary; she was bold, valued process, and cultivated collegiality. In this paper, the authors examine these qualities, which they seek to emulate, and which contribute to excellence in social work practice. Examples from Roselle and the authors' practice are used to illustrate these behaviors. *[Article copies available for a fee from The Haworth Document Delivery Service: 1-800-HAWORTH. E-mail address: <docdelivery@haworthpress.com> Website: <http://www.HaworthPress.com> © 2006 by The Haworth Press, Inc. All rights reserved.]*

KEYWORDS. Use of self, professional use of self, being bold, valuing process, staying in the mess, colleague, collegiality

One of the authors was posthumously visited by Professor Roselle Kurland in her sleep:

The authors wish to thank Andy Malekoff for not taking "No" for an answer when they thought they would not be able to write this paper. Keren Ludwig thanks Lisa Bilander Gray for making her aware of social group work practice and for introducing her to Roselle Kurland.

[Haworth co-indexing entry note]: "On Being Bold, Valuing Process, and Cultivating Collegiality." Ludwig, Keren, and Priska Imberti. Co-published simultaneously in *Social Work with Groups* (The Haworth Press, Inc.) Vol. 29, No. 2/3, 2006, pp. 47-55; and: *Making Joyful Noise: The Art, Science, and Soul of Group Work* (ed: Andrew Malekoff, Robert Salmon, and Dominique Moyse Steinberg) The Haworth Press, Inc., 2006, pp. 47-55. Single or multiple copies of this article are available for a fee from The Haworth Document Delivery Service [1-800-HAWORTH, 9:00 a.m. - 5:00 p.m. (EST). E-mail address: docdelivery@haworth press.com].

I walk into the back of a classroom. The students have their chairs in a semi-circle with their backs facing me. Roselle is in the middle of the circle and is talking with the students about their groups. Roselle is very engaged; she waves her hands and, as she speaks, her voice rises and falls to punctuate the details. She might be talking about "equifinality" or "staying in the mess." I am thrilled to see this. This is what I have been longing to experience with her again. Suddenly I am struck by the ephemeral nature of this life-after-death teaching moment and I start to cry. Roselle looks up and, without distracting her students, she shushes me. Then, in a half whisper, and with a smile, Roselle tells me to keep the fact that she is dead to myself. Roselle returns to teach the students and I watch.

Roselle's message to us is that it is still possible to pass on her vibrant legacy, and that in her teachings, she is alive. Her message, teaching, and writing are gifts that she leaves to all of us. We can share these gifts with others even if we never knew her. We feel this is her mandate.

Having said that, Roselle did write volumes but there are three very unique lessons that she gave through her "use of self," which we aim to emulate and would like to share in this paper. They are: being bold, valuing process, and cultivating collegiality. These purposeful uses of self will be explored and illustrated with examples from our own and Roselle's practice.

Use of self, or professional use of self, are terms often referred to but rarely defined. In this paper, the act of using the self can be understood as the following:

> [a worker] is aware of himself as an agent, aware of self as personally involved, aware of the need to discipline the personal involvement, and is able to own and maintain awareness of the self and professional self, making conscious use of the latter. (p. 21, William Rosenthal as summarized by Lewis, 1991)

In addition to being aware of reactions and selective about which to demonstrate or act on, Lewis (1991) adds that as an educator, his conscious use of self helped students achieve learning goals. This is definitely something that we saw in Roselle and an aspect of her that we try to internalize. In our practice, conscious use of self facilitates our being available to clients, our ability to make institutional change, and to work effectively with peers, supervisors, and supervisees.

BEING BOLD

"Be bold!" said Roselle, "Just say it!" If and when we would complain about our internships, jobs, or even a policy we disliked, Roselle would listen but also direct us to take the complaint back to whom it belonged. This is not easy.

As workers, we know what is right and just for our clients. Yet we also know that the environments we find ourselves in may not always be hospitable to client needs. We know that when we express ourselves we may face consequences ranging from dirty looks to putting our jobs in jeopardy. Being bold means that it is better to express oneself and face the consequences than to be only half a social worker, an automaton, or a bureaucratic rubber-stamper. Yet workers know that to survive agency life they must choose battles wisely. We often wonder if Roselle the worker was as bold as Roselle the professor. Since she has died we feel that we must be even bolder because she is no longer here to debate whether a particular situation calls for boldness or not. The following is an example of one of us deciding to be bold:

> As a school-based Spanish-speaking social worker, I was recently sought out by Elena, a twelve-year-old immigrant from Central America. Elena spoke no English and showed a speech delay in Spanish that had yet to be diagnosed by the school. The school district had taken the stance that a monolingual, immersion-based English language environment would best help immigrant students learn English. Elena approached me and said, "I want to borrow books from the school library but I don't know how to and I don't know where the library is." I took Elena to the library and helped her to register for borrowing privileges. Elena asked for a book in Spanish or a bi-lingual book. I translated this request to the librarian who responded that she had been "strongly encouraged" by the district not to stock any foreign language books. The librarian offered Elena some picture books with no words at all. These books were meant for babies. I felt this was a moment that called for boldness and told the librarian, "Well, I would like to take you and 'the district' to China with no knowledge of the Mandarin language and immerse you into the culture without any signs or anything at all to help you. Let's see how well you do!" I pursued the matter further and discovered that there is a library in the district with foreign language books. The librarian has agreed to bring

them to our library through inter-library loan, and they are now available to Elena.

Being bold means recognizing that we have something to say and that there is no one else who is responsible to say it for us. It also means that we take a strong stance and own it. In the above example, the worker took a strong stance and advocated for the student. She also communicated that the librarian was responsible to advocate for the needs of children rather than serving the district's mandate. The worker made a demand that the librarian be bold as well.

In "Not Just One of the Gang . . ." (1993) Roselle and Robert Salmon have written of the importance of teachers and supervisors modeling behavior for students:

> Since students will, to some extent, model themselves after the teachers they respect, perhaps one of the most important characteristics for the teacher is that of passion–passion for the subject and learning to be connected to the work with clients. (p. 166)

When Roselle was bold she effectively modeled passion; wild horses could not get her to be silent on an issue she cared about. The effect of Roselle's boldness was paradoxical. On the one hand it meant that it was not always easy to be with her because she held us accountable in ways that could feel uncomfortable. At the same time, one could always be sure of how she felt, which made for a very secure feeling.

Roselle was clear about wanting to be "challenging with an arm around the shoulder" and she blended these things well. There is an art in this: she challenged the things we said or did while supporting us as people. She did not analyze us or diagnose us with pervasive or fatal personality flaws. Since she never held anything back, including the times that she celebrated us, we could be confident that we knew how she felt in the moment.

VALUING PROCESS

Valuing process is something Roselle would refer to often when she spoke of "staying in the mess." This means that she was less interested in outcome than she was in truly grappling and engaging with the matter at hand. Roselle's interest in "the mess" was made very clear in her and Robert Salmon's elaboration of John Dewey's problem solving approach (1910) in which step three–exploration of the problem–is given most page space:

> The problem is explored. As it is explored, additional information may be gathered from the individual about the situation. Group members need to really listen to what the individual is saying. They may ask questions about the problem and about the feelings of the individual. As they listen and question and come to understand the problem through the eyes of the individual who has raised it, they develop empathy and communicate that along with their understanding, concern, caring and support. (p. 9, 1992)

When we spoke with Roselle she would put this third step into practice. She would ask us questions to help her, and us, to really parse out what we had in mind. She would not accept platitudes or jargon; she needed to know exactly what we meant. In exploring and seeking to deeply understand what we had to say, and by telling us directly to do so, she demanded that we "be specific!"

This process oriented, non-judgmental stance was very alien for many of us who studied with her. One of the authors was particularly moved:

> I grew up in an environment that valued outcomes and accomplishments; particularly in higher education. I never felt I could measure up to what was expected of me in this arena. Being given permission to struggle was miraculous for me because so much of my time was spent doing just that.

Roselle's valuing of process made it easier for us to really open up our practice to her, and our own, examination. This is a gift we retain today. It allows us to become better workers.

The authors try to replicate this stance in their own practice and extend it to others. One of the authors reflects on her role as a new field instructor:

> I am a field instructor to a student for the first time and I have been thinking about the fact that I have very high expectations of her. When I consider these expectations I realize that my hope is not for her to perform or to "get it right." Rather, my wish is for her is to fully engage in the struggles inherent in learning to be a social

worker and discovering new and genuine ways of interacting with people.

One of the ways the author encourages the student to be in touch with her struggles is through modeling that it is okay to do so. The author is transparent about her own faults and struggles while also showing competence, confidence, and ability.

Being transparent about strengths and faults was something that Roselle did. She had no problem taking credit for what she knew and what she could do. She was open about her shortcomings as well. This quality is illustrated by the following vignette that comes from a class designed to help students write scholarly articles:

> A student decided to write about the psychosocial effects of lipodystrophy and social work intervention with those who experience it. Lipodystrophy refers to physical changes in the bodies of people taking a particular set of HIV medications. This student wanted to use his own experience of lipodystrophy, particularly the radical transformation of his face, as a way to connect the reader to the experience. When he presented this in class, Roselle talked about how important it was for workers to share their experiences. She also said to the student, "You know when we first discussed this privately in my office, I had difficulty sitting with it. The first thing I said to you was 'I don't see what you are talking about. I would never know you had HIV if you didn't tell me. There is nothing wrong with your face.' I think I was rushing to solutions because it was hard for me to stay in the mess."

Hearing that an admired professor struggled in this way was profound. It let us know that having difficulty with the painful things others faced was normal and that if we failed to stay in the mess with them we could own up to it and come back to it again. Roselle showed, by example, that we all have ordinarily faulty and extraordinary parts of ourselves. They co-exist together and we use them as workers–whether we like it or not.

COLLEGIALITY

Roselle once complimented the authors on their collegial relationship saying: "You can have classmates, you can have friends, but to have a colleague is very rare." Elsewhere, writing with her colleague Andrew Malekoff, they have written:

> We need to seek out and then value true colleagues–those who will listen, understand, share, accept, challenge, affirm, validate, support, disagree, respect. . . . True colleagues are, indeed, rare. We need them. We need to seek them out. And when we find them, we need to treasure them. And in the work that we do, that is so very demanding, difficult, moving and special, we also need to be real colleagues to others. (2002, pp. 6-7)

The authors consider themselves to be colleagues. This is so in spite of the multiple differences between them. Like Kurland and Malekoff (2002), one of us lives in Long Island and the other in New York City. One of us loves to converse by e-mail while the other can't stand it and prefers the telephone. One of us is casual and the other formal. One of us is romantic and long-winded (or thorough), the other is neurotic and curt (or to the point). In spite of these differences, we experience that, like a group, the whole of us is bigger than the sum of our parts. As a team, we can accomplish things that we cannot do apart. It is also more fun for us and takes some of the agony out of things like writing or putting ideas together for presentation. Yet at times, the agony is increased because we have to confront disagreements with each other. We rely on our history and track record together at these challenging times to help us put forth our best efforts and give each other the benefit of the doubt.

The authors find that the most basic ingredient of their collegiality is a generosity of spirit. This means first and foremost being generous with time; time on the phone, time on the dreaded e-mail, time on the Long Island Rail Road, time on the Brooklyn Queens Expressway, time at conferences, time with each other's families and time at the mall or at the movies. Like all other social workers, we are busy but we have made a conscious choice to invest in each other and ourselves by nurturing our relationship with time. Being able to "accept, challenge . . . [and] disagree . . ." (Kurland and Malekoff, 2002, p. 6) is not easy, but these aspects of a relationship will never develop if they are not fed by the gift of time.

Another way we see generosity of spirit being important is in flexibility of roles and a willingness to accept criticism. We are in awe of all that Robert Salmon and Roselle Kurland have done together as partners in terms of writing and being leaders in the field of social work with groups. We have always been very interested in the nitty-gritty of their partnership which spanned many years. We would often ask Roselle questions like–how did you meet Bob? where did the ideas come from? how did you write? One day Roselle told us the following story:

> Bob and I always wrote separately but at one time he wanted to write together. I thought this would be very difficult but I said okay and he came to my office at the appointed time with a notebook and a well-sharpened pencil. Bob and I talked and then he wrote down some things in his [imagine her voice start to groan] very big long handwriting [Roselle had short concise handwriting]. He showed it to me and I said, "Bob, that sucks!" Bob was unfazed. He said "Okay," crumpled up the page, and we started again.

We like this story for many reasons–not the least of which is the fact that they wrote on paper with pencils! This story shows how Bob and Roselle were different from each other, that they accommodated the differences by being flexible, how they checked ego at the door in order to work and how they each put their best foot forward. It also shows a very pedestrian moment in their partnership. We find this very encouraging because the bulk of our experience is composed of pedestrian or mundane moments (the deadline for this paper is soon and we have nothing! . . . remember that you have to justify the abstract . . . how do I get to the BQE from here?) As seen in the example above, having these moments and struggling to create does not preclude the achievement of the beauty and genius to which we aspire to.

CONCLUSIONS

Group workers are unique in that they know that every moment is significant. We do not distinguish between exalted "clinical" moments and mundane moments with clients in our practice. We know that every moment is important; we don't need to be sitting in a circle, staring into each others eyes and passing a tissue box for the group to have started. The group starts when the doorbell rings and in the waiting room.

Conscious use of self then is especially important to group workers because it is something we benefit from practicing all of the time. Roselle had much to offer us in terms of modeling practices that we can make use of in our own work. By being bold she was authentically herself, by valuing process she was able to truly connect to others, and in cultivating collegiality she was able to relish her professional life and accomplish much more than she would have alone. Having put this on paper we hope that this teaching of hers can be incorporated into the work of other social workers–even those who never knew her. In our work, we are conscious of being bold, valuing process and cultivating collegiality first and foremost because they are good practices. In addition, when we practice this way, in our hearts, Roselle continues to be alive.

REFERENCES

Dewey, J. (1910). *How we think*. Boston: Heath.

Kurland, R. and Salmon, R. (1992). Group work vs. case work in a group. *Social Work with Groups*, 15(4), 3-14.

Kurland, R. and Salmon, R. (1993). Not just one of the gang: Group workers and their role as an authority. *Social Work with Groups*, 16(1/2), 153-167.

Kurland, R. and Malekoff, A. (2002). Introduction. *Social Work with Groups*, 25(1/2), 1-7.

Lewis, H. (1991). Teacher's style and use of professional self in social work education. *Journal of Teaching in Social Work*, 5(2), 17-29.

Putting Ideas to Paper:
A Guideline for Practitioners (and Others)
Who Wish to Write for Publication

Andrew Malekoff

SUMMARY. This article offers guidelines for aspiring writers who wish to have their work published. Especially geared for practitioners, it includes suggestions for getting started, staying focused, structuring an article, understanding the writing process, overcoming frustration, coping with reviewers' critiques and enduring through to completion. *[Article copies available for a fee from The Haworth Document Delivery Service: 1-800-HAWORTH. E-mail address: <docdelivery@haworthpress.com> Website: <http://www.HaworthPress.com> © 2006 by The Haworth Press, Inc. All rights reserved.]*

KEYWORDS. Writing, publication, group work, social work, professional journal

INTRODUCTION

When Roselle Kurland and I became editors of *Social Work with Groups* in 1990, one thing that we quickly agreed upon was the need to encourage practitioners to write for the Journal. What "encourage" meant to us was to provide more than inspiration. It meant offering practical advice and ongoing support for aspiring writers. We did this by: (1) In-

[Haworth co-indexing entry note]: "Putting Ideas to Paper: A Guideline for Practitioners (and Others) Who Wish to Write for Publication." Malekoff, Andrew. Co-published simultaneously in *Social Work with Groups* (The Haworth Press, Inc.) Vol. 29, No. 2/3, 2006, pp. 57-72; and: *Making Joyful Noise: The Art, Science, and Soul of Group Work* (ed: Andrew Malekoff, Robert Salmon, and Dominique Moyse Steinberg) The Haworth Press, Inc., 2006, pp. 57-72. Single or multiple copies of this article are available for a fee from The Haworth Document Delivery Service [1-800-HAWORTH, 9:00 a.m. - 5:00 p.m. (EST). E-mail address: docdelivery@haworthpress.com].

corporating guidelines about writing in our "From the Editor" commentaries that appeared in the beginning of each journal issue, (2) Offering detailed recommendations for revising promising manuscripts that were not accepted for publication on the first try, (3) Developing and presenting a workshop on writing for publication that we called "Putting Ideas to Paper," and (4) Reaching out and appealing to practitioners and students and helping them to identify themes for writing.

I am not certain what our success rate was in encouraging new authors, but it pleased us immensely when someone who we recruited or encouraged to write did so successfully. Roselle Kurland died suddenly and unexpectedly on June 7, 2005. As editor of the Journal I carry the legacy that was begun by both of us. This article represents a distillation of the ideas and concepts that we presented in our workshops and editorials on writing, and that were a part of our private conversations over fifteen years of working together. As such, my name appears as author of the article; however, Roselle's spirit is with me in every step of the writing.

Normally, we asked writers who submitted manuscripts written in first person, to change their articles to third person except when presenting practice illustrations. For the purposes of this article I am defying our own rule and writing and speaking to you, my reader, directly.

PUBLISH TO PRESERVE

For me, writing always begins with a desire to capture an experience or an idea and then pass it on, share it, make it available to others. In other words–to preserve it. The well-known slogan that I have heard repeated by colleagues who teach in universities is "publish or perish," referring to the relationship between published works and job security (tenure) and advancement (promotion). Of course every job has its special demands. How sad for those in academia where the "publish or perish" sword is the primary motivating force, although I know many for whom that is not the case.

An alternative slogan that I coined for myself is "publish to preserve." My fellow editor and friend, the late Howard Goldstein (1998), said, "writing is an act of creating a virtual reality. It is an intimately personal attempt to transform an idea–what is in your mind and often in your heart–into a coherent and informative account of what you want to tell" (p. 452). Writing, for me, usually starts with a personal practice experience or one that a colleague shares with me. It is usually something that moves me or illuminates a concept or practice approach. What is the first thing that any of us does after a moving or frustrating practice experience? If you are like me, you tell someone, you tell the story of what happened, often in a state of excitement, passion, or sometimes despair.

Telling the story of what happened in practice is one way to preserve it. But, as fresh as the story is when we first tell it and when it is closest to the moment that it happens, even the best of stories have a way of fading in time. The memory fades and the emotions tied to it dissipate. Not always. I remember someone once remarking that if you don't get it down on paper and only tell it, that it is like trying to nail whispers to the wall. So, to get started, it always helps me to write the story down as I might tell it to someone in all of its raw and unvarnished glory. I save the editing for much later. I urge you to just get it down on paper.[1]

To best capture the moment, write it down when it is most fresh in your mind. Or, if you prefer, audio tape the story and transcribe it. Sometimes, I am told, "But I just can't seem to get started." One suggestion that has helped is to write it down in the form of a letter that you are writing to a good friend or colleague. For example, "Dear Margaret, You will not believe what happened last night in my 'single mothers' group.' It was so moving that I just have to tell someone. So I chose you . . ." Writing a letter, a lost art, to someone close to you can have a meandering and conversational quality to it that is less inhibiting than more formal professional writing. The personal connection to the receiver provides a writer greater freedom and less a feeling of being judged by critics. I find that it is a good way to get started, to get off the dime.

Start by telling your story, getting it down on paper. Later on you can think about the moral of the story; what ideas and concepts the story illustrates that can be used to teach others. Regarding writing to preserve, Ruth Middleman once told me, "You cannot sit on knowledge . . . not to preserve an experience is to betray it."

Publish to preserve!

NUTS AND BOLTS

Beyond slogans and motivation to get started and get going, it is helpful to have a framework or an outline for writing an article for publication. Not every published article is formatted in exactly the same way. Sometimes an unconventional structure or style works and finds its way to print. Some editors and publishers are flexible in this way, others are more rigid. Nevertheless, most articles–unless they are written as essays, commentary, or as special features that a journal might invite–include a standard set of elements. The following annotated framework provides a useful outline and suggested page lengths.

I. STATEMENT OF THE ISSUE AND ITS SIGNIFICANCE (1-2 PAGES)

It should come from practice or a personal experience. By the second or third paragraph you should state the purpose of the article by saying: "This article will . . ." or "It aims to . . ." For example, "This article will provide group work practitioners with a framework for planning, implementing, and evaluating groups for children who, after losing a parent in the aftermath of a terrorist attack, are experiencing trauma and complicated grief . . ."

II. REVIEW OF THE LITERATURE (3-5 PAGES)

This is *your* statement about the state of the literature on the subject or topic. You need to write this by focusing on ideas or concepts in the literature related to the subject and how to make sense of it. You can use an historical approach (i.e., when your theme was first introduced, to present time) or contemporaneous approach (i.e., "Some of the most significant themes on this subject are . . .") to reviewing the literature.

The idea of a literature review is not to quote everyone who ever had anything to say about the theme of your article. That takes your voice out of the mix. Rather, be selective in choosing to include others who have written about the subject to help amplify your voice. Write about what you have learned about the subject, what you know, and what you think exists in the literature that will be interesting and helpful to others. Use quotes sparingly and selectively to enhance *your* message, not to obscure it with what others have to say. Remember, this is *your* article.

Think of the literature review as a conversation. Address what you think about what others have said versus regurgitating the literature itself. The idea is not to simply include everything you can find on the subject and dispassionately summarize everyone else's work. Rather, tell your reader why what you cite is important to you–to your way of viewing things–and why it turns you on. When incorporating citations into your text, think of them as notations to help the reader know where to go to get more information about that issue, idea, or person. Having empathy with your readers will help you to identify what areas they might like to explore in greater depth and which authors they might want to get to know better.

As my colleague Dominique Moyse Steinberg (2005) advises her students about preparing a review of the literature, "Your heartbeat should both be evident and drive the conversation."

Finally, use subheadings to organize your review of the literature (and the rest of your article). Readers will more easily follow and integrate concepts and ideas when organized in related parts that each has good transitional sentences that carry them from section to section.

III. PRESENTATION OF "DATA" AND DISCUSSION (7-10 PAGES)

This is organized by ideas versus a meandering description. You need to add structure to the presentation of your experience. For example, it is most helpful to use a number, i.e., "There are five major interventions . . ." or "The framework to be presented has four key components . . ." Numbering gives authority to what you are writing.

The concepts that help to organize your manuscript usually emerge from one of two directions:

1. **Inductive.** *You have a powerful story and want to tell the story. Okay, do that and tell the readers what the concepts it demonstrates are.* This applies to a program description and practice illustrations. The description and illustrations cannot stand alone in a scholarly journal. They must be punctuated and supported by a presentation of concepts that under gird the narrative presentation. Using concepts to support illustrations is also a great way to help to organize and structure your manuscript with subheadings.

2. **Deductive.** *You have an idea about something, practice concepts you wish to advance and you want to illustrate it, bring it to life for the reader.* A theoretical or conceptual presentation is only as strong as the illustrations that make the concepts and theory real for the reader. A good paper will bring the thinking and doing (and feeling) together by integrating the conceptual with the practical in the form of vivid practice illustrations that demonstrate the theory in action and, in some cases, the practitioner's feelings and motivations behind their conceptually-based interventions.

It is important to emphasize that sometimes manuscripts that are submitted for consideration include beautiful process of practice and no concepts. Others include extensive discussion of theory and concepts but meager one-sentence descriptions or illustrations. Articles must blend the two—concepts and description. Following is an excerpt from an editorial that Roselle and I wrote and that appeared in the first volume of the Journal that we edited together (Kurland and Malekoff, 1992).

> Broadly speaking, two kinds of articles about direct practice are most prevalent among those not accepted for publication in the journal. First, there are articles that describe the needs and dynamics of a particular population group—those who have been abused or persons with a particular illness, for example. While such delineations are often informative, too frequently the reference to groups and group work practice in such articles is minimal and seems to be appended reluctantly and uneasily to qualify the article for consideration in this, a journal on work with groups. The portions of such articles that refer to group work practice are not an integral part of the authors' presentations and seem artificial.
>
> Second, there are articles that describe a group and its process, be it a particular kind of group or a group with a particular population, with which the author worked. While such descriptions are often interesting, too frequently their purpose is unclear. In these articles, the practice described is not examined conceptually and therefore the applicability to other groups of the work depicted is never made clear. Given the complexity of groups, of individuals, and of situations, articles that are *solely* descriptive, that do not look critically or analytically at work that is being presented, are not helpful to their readers.
>
> With respect to both kinds of papers, population-oriented or purely descriptive, we have found practice illustrations to be too general to capture the essence of the work described. Illustrations that capture the true nature of the group, bringing to life the interaction among the members and between the members and the worker are too often absent.
>
> What we would like to see included in *Social Work with Groups* are articles that bring together the doing and thinking of group work prac-

tice. In articles that emphasize knowledge of the needs of a particular population, implications for and illustrations of group work practice based on such knowledge need to be integral. In articles that portray practice through the presentation of descriptive vignettes and examples, the rationale that underpins the practice, the thinking behind it, and the implications for future practice with groups is crucial elements. (pp. 1-2)

IV. CONCLUSIONS AND IMPLICATIONS (1-2 PAGES)

As you come to an end you want help the reader to look ahead. To give authority to your work, make bold statements about what you have presented. Roselle's students are often fond of recalling one of her directives. She always told her students, "Be bold!" Sometimes writers are afraid and say, "What if someone else wrote about it." Some writers feel the need to start every paragraph with everyone else's ideas and theirs' at the end. Flip it around. Tell yourself that this is your paper. Have confidence in it. Don't be afraid or timid that someone will say that you don't know what you are talking about. Don't start every sentence tentatively with "It seems . . ." or "Maybe . . ." or "Perhaps . . ." That is too soft. BE BOLD.

V. REFERENCES

Most journals have an "information for authors" section printed in the journal itself or that can be requested or accessed over the Internet. Instructions for authors provide instructions for style, including a format for how references are to be listed.

ON ENDURANCE

Getting it down on paper, having a framework and being bold are helpful. However, the actual process of writing is not quite as linear as the outline just presented, nor is it propelled solely by an attitude of confidence. I truly believe that the essence of good writing is rewriting. If you don't know that–don't know how good writing evolves and how many drafts it can take to get a decent manuscript–it can be a demoralizing process. In an attempt to deconstruct the process is a poem, a guideline, a movie review and one writer's experience of the writing process.

Poetry

I wrote this poem for our writing workshops. Because it was first presented at a workshop we offered in Denver, Colorado I called it "rocky mountain writer's workshop" (Malekoff, 1999b). I later discovered that Roselle used this in her professional seminar class in which students were expected to write high-level articles.

rocky mountain writer's workshop

i have an idea
i write a sentence
i crumple the page.
i have an idea
i write a sentence
i crumple the page.
i have an idea
i write a sentence
i crumple the page.
i have an idea
i write a sentence
i crumple the page.

i live on
a mountain of crumpled pages;

an avalanche of aborted ideas
blanket me.

there is only one way out:

i have an idea
i write a sentence.

Writing is a craft, a precision skill that is not easily mastered (Zinsser, 1998). In his book, *The Tenant* one of Bernard Malamud's (1971) characters, writer Willie Spearmint says that "Writing down words is like hitting the paper with a one ton hammer" (p. 34). Although not indispensable, a guideline might help.

Guideline

This is a distillation of feedback that Roselle and I often gave to authors after reviewing manuscripts. It takes the outline presented above a little further (Kurland and Malekoff, 1997).

1. Begin with a clear understanding of a few major themes (two to five) you want to cover, a few major points you want to make.
2. Develop an outline with tentative subheadings to help you organize the paper.
3. Write an introduction that clearly describes the importance of the paper and its purpose.
4. Illustrate conceptually oriented papers with practice descriptions.
5. Punctuate practice-oriented descriptions with organizing concepts and principles.
6. Write a brief conclusion to summarize and lend closure to your presentation.
7. Anticipate having to write a few drafts before you begin to see your work take shape.
8. Look at other articles, not only for content, but also for style and structure.
9. Ask someone you can trust to give you honest feedback about your manuscript.
10. If necessary, ask someone with writing skill, be it a colleague or a friend, to help you edit your work.
11. Await your response with the idea that a rejection need not mean the end of the work.
12. Carefully consider the reviewers' comments and go back to the drawing board (pp. 2-3).

Hands on a Hardbody

One of my favorite all time documentary movies is entitled, "Hands on a Hardbody" (1998). Filmed by S. R. Bindler, it is about a contest that takes place each year at a Nissan dealership in Longview, Texas. Twenty-three names are drawn at random and this group gets the opportunity to participate. One reviewer (Brown, 2005) describes how it works.

The rules are as follows: one hand must remain on the truck at all times; no leaning or squatting allowed; if the hand is raised even momentarily, the contestant is out. One five-minute break is permitted every hour, and one 15-minute break every six hours. The last three survivors–excuse us, contestants–must be tested for drugs. The results are hilarious. The gloves irritate hands (sweat could ruin the truck's finish), legs go numb, people get on each other's nerves. Strategy is involved, cheaters are accused, competition is fierce. 'It's a contest, they say, of stamina, but it's who can maintain their sanity the longest,' we're told by 1992 winner Benny Perkins, who competes once again . . . Each contestant represents something, but which will win out: desperation (a woman tired of riding her bike everywhere but who can't afford car payments), determination (a toothless woman who "tr[ies] to finish everything I start"), God (a woman's church holds a prayer chain for her as she communes with Jesus by the truck), endurance (a former Marine who once stayed awake for five days), or experience (Perkins is sure he knows all the tricks)?

Viewing this film for the first time, it reminded me throughout of my own experience of writing for publication, stamina and maintaining one's sanity. Keeping one hand on the truck at all times . . . pencil to paper . . . fingers to keyboard . . . staying with it . . . enduring.

One Writer's Experience of the Writing Process

I remember seeing and enjoying another movie, "Finding Forester," about a writing-legend-turned-recluse and the friendship he develops with an inner-city teenage boy that he mentors. He tells him, "Write the first draft from your heart . . . write the second draft from your head." And a little later in their developing relationship he advises, "The best moment is when you have read your best draft and before they tear it down."

It took me many years to discover a method to my own writing (if you can call it that), a process that included an integration of thoughts, actions and feelings. Following is a summary of that process (Malekoff, 1999a).

1. I begin with an idea that excites me, turns me on.
2. I spend hours, sometimes days, agonizing over the first sentence or paragraph.

3. I write a stream of consciousness draft that is embarrassing at best, psychotic at worst.
4. I let the draft sit for days, dreading a return to what I feel is an incomprehensible mess.
5. I go back to the draft and try to fix it, to clean up the mess.
6. I agonize over a second draft, convinced that nothing will come of it.
7. I put it aside again, the second draft feeling no better than the first.
8. I stay away from the draft for days, hoping to return with fresh eyes.
9. I go back and agonize some more.
10. Sometimes I ask someone to read it, hoping they will lie and say, "it's not that bad."
11. I realize that anyone who tells me it is okay is not being honest.
12. I try to find an honest critic even though a part of me doesn't want to hear from them because it always means more work for me and having to deal with criticism.
13. After an honest critique, I read it over and let it sit some more.
14. I go back and edit the undifferentiated mass, chipping away here and modifying there.
15. If I am fortunate there is a glimmer of hope.
16. When there is hope I go back to the draft sooner and with greater anticipation.
17. It starts to make sense and, for the first time in the process, a joyful feeling emerges, if ever so slightly.
18. I cannot stay away from the manuscript and feel compelled to write and edit until it is just right. This is my favorite phase of the process.
19. I am satisfied.
20. I give it to an honest critic, convinced that they will say it is perfect.
21. They tell me it needs more work.
22. I feel angry. Tired of the process, I don't want to do anymore.
23. I go back to it, consider the critique and roll up my sleeves. Again.
24. I am finished.

This is a reasonable facsimile of the process. It is not always exactly like this. Sometimes it is easier. Thoughts and feelings flow more smoothly and I am able to move more gracefully and rapidly through the process. Most often, though, the process is uncomfortable, awkward, annoying and painful. The joyful and energizing part (#18) is usually short-lived and intensely pleasurable. There is nothing else I would rather be doing at this stage of writing. The relief of finishing is brief, particularly when the goal is to get what I write published. There is always the risk that no one will accept what I submit for publication and the possibility that my effort will be trashed.

On Rejection

> I found this paper to be vague, confused, ambiguous, and poorly defined . . . not really innovative. The author wanders around blindly and presents a confused description of the designated actions involved. The organization is very poor, the paper lacks continuity, and if there is a clear purpose, it is not clearly established. The author uses vague and gimmicky terms. The paper never arrives at its undeclared destination and I doubt that many passengers will feel that the trip was worthwhile. I see this as a paper that would not contribute anything.

This is an actual critique of a manuscript I submitted for publication to another journal. It was hard to swallow. I wrote a poem about it, to capture what it felt like to read such words about something that I invested my blood, sweat, and tears into. The reviewer's comments are repeated, in *italics*. In **bold,** is a recounting of my immediate interpretation of the critique.

I found the paper [by Malekoff] to be:

Vague, confused, ambiguous, and poorly defined
    jack-ass;
Not really innovative
    boring-clod;
The author wanders around blindly
    listless-fool;
The organization is very poor
    awkward-klutz;
The paper lacks continuity
    scatter-brain;
If there is a clear purpose, it is not clearly established
    aim-less;

The author uses vague and gimmicky terms
  no-depth-dufus;
The paper never arrives at its undeclared destination
  no-vision-vermin;
I doubt many passengers will feel that the trip was worthwhile
  worthless-wanker;
I see this as a paper that would not contribute anything
  ze-ro.

Of course, if I am to go any further after reading a critique of my work I must get beyond personalizing the commentary and try to look, with a critical eye, at what needs to be improved. The trouble is that some reviewers tend to attack rather than critique. Having been on the receiving end of brutal attacks on my writing, I have made a personal pledge as an editor never to send such a review to a writer. I may send a highly detailed and constructive critique that will be difficult for a writer to absorb; however, I am always careful to try not to stand on a soapbox and discourage writers.

An illustration of a direct critique, with no punches pulled about my writing came from Ruth Middleman, whom I asked to review a draft of book chapter I was writing on the use of activities in groups. Here is what she wrote to me: ". . . My main reaction is that you kill through quotes to the point where they become meaningless. It's as if you have to have some other person say something before it is valuable. In the meantime, what do you believe is your purpose and use of activities?" This was not easy for me to read at first. But it was *right on*. It is the kind of comment that stung at first, but that has stuck with me and benefited me for years. Compare this with the earlier critique. Both stung and one helped while the other only hurt.

When Roselle and I facilitated workshops on writing we asked participants to identify obstacles to writing. They were typically divided into five categories:

- logistics of writing (space, time, interruptions);
- technical concerns (style, too much to say, use of language);
- existential aspects of writing (loneliness);
- motivation (procrastination, feeling intimidated, lack self confidence); and
- rejection (exposure, fear of failure, and embarrassment).

In writing for publication you must know and come to accept that rejection comes with the territory and although any rejection is painful and even the most thoughtful critique will sting, sometimes they come in a particularly disturbing dose as illustrated above. According to William Zinsser (1998) in his excellent book, *On writing well: The classic guide to writing nonfiction*, writing is about craft (mastering a precise skill) and about attitude (how you use the skill to express your personality). Zinsser's book is a great companion for aspiring and practicing writers. Some of his suggestions relate to the obstacles listed above and address both emotional and technical dimensions of writing.

- Style is tied to psyche, and writing has deep psychological roots (p. 22).
- Perhaps [a writer's] style won't solidify for years as your style, your voice. Just as it takes time to find yourself as a person, it takes time to find yourself as a stylist and even then your style will change as your grow older (p. 26).
- Never say anything in writing that you wouldn't comfortably say in conversation (p. 27).
- Hear how the words sound. Readers read with their eyes but hear the words. Consider writing by ear (p. 36).
- Writing is visual. Shorter paragraphs are more inviting (p. 80).
- Write with authority. Don't use qualifiers, be bold (pp. 71-72).
- Rewriting is the essence of writing well (p. 84).

I add to this list of sage advice, Goldstein's reflection (1998) on good writing as it pertains to a social work readership.

- Most important, good writing enhances our knowledge and understanding of the human conditions that concern social work, thereby strengthening our identity, function, and purpose (p. 454).

On Acceptance

Receiving an acceptance letter for a manuscript that has been toiled over is one of the most professionally uplifting experiences one can experience. This is especially so in the early going–when your first article is accepted. It is a cause for celebration and sharing. Don't be modest. Get the word out. After all, your contribution is intended to enhance the field. Don't be shy about a little self-promotion. If you find a journal that likes "your stuff," and where you feel there is a good match, don't hesitate to go back to them. In time, try your hand at other journals, spread your wings.

The best compliment I can receive is when someone who teaches tells me that their students like something that I have written and have included it in their practice logs or papers. Sometimes a colleague in a university will send me a copy. If you are a professor you should know that writers, at least this one, loves it when you share this information about what we have written. It is encouraging.

Feel great about your published article. Celebrate. Then come back down to earth and expect to face more scrutiny as you forge ahead with your next article. Practice makes better, but it does not ensure acceptance and, as the process described above details, there is always hard work ahead no matter how accomplished a writer one becomes.

On Synergy

For me, the logistical obstacle of not having the time to write is best addressed by embracing the concept of "synergy." If you can make a conscious and real connection between what you are writing and its present benefit to parts of your work life and personal development, it will not be experienced as "something extra to do that I don't have the time for." Whenever I make a decision to write something I tie it to a workshop that I might present, a proposal for funding that I might write, an issue in supervision that I might address with a staff member, or an intervention for direct practice that I might wish to master, for example.

The concept of synergy, the simultaneous action of different parts, allows me to see the time spent writing as time well spent, time that will pay multiple and long lasting dividends whether or not what I write is accepted for publication now or later or never at all. The process is the payoff, as well as the product. And, if the product does not please the reviewers, I can try again. And, if I choose not to I can use the material I created for something new and different at some other time. What I write is never wasted. Someone else's rejection of my work is *never* the end of the road. What I write is always conserved and sometimes recycled for later use. And every time I write it makes me into a better writer as I continue the process of empathizing with my readers, trying to feel and think what they might feel and think as they read my words. And, when I am confident that they will see and feel what I do, and that they might be inspired and educated and maybe even moved in the process, then I will know that I have succeeded.

Write on!

NOTE

1. Of course, practice illustrations used for publication should be adequately disguised.

REFERENCES

Bindler, S.R. (1999). *Hands on a hard body* (documentary video). New York: Ideal Enterprises.

Brown, J. (2005). Hands on a Hardbody review published on Amazon.com viewed on August 11, http://www.amazon.com/exec/obidos/tg/detail/-/B00000JYWY/002-4895182-8043203?v=glance

Goldstein, H. (1998). On writing for publication. *Families in Society*, 79:5, 451-454.

Kurland, R. and Malekoff, A. (1992). From the editors. *Social Work with Groups*, 15:4, 1-2.

Kurland, R. and Malekoff, A. (1997). From the editors. *Social Work with Groups, 20:1, 1-3.*

Malamud, B. (1971). *The tenant.* New York: Farrar, Straus, and Giroux.

Malekoff, A. (1999a). A practitioner's journey to becoming a writer. *Families in Society*, 80:2, 190-194. (This essay also appeared in *Social Work with Groups*, 1999, 22:1, 7-11).

Malekoff, A. (1999b). *Rocky mountain writer's workshop* (poetry). Presented at the 21st Annual Symposium of the Association for the Advancement of Social Work with Groups, Denver, Colorado, October 22.

Zinsser, W. (1998). *On writing well: The classic guide to writing nonfiction* (6th edition). New York: HarperCollins.

Education for the Group Worker's Reality: The Special Qualities and World View of Those Drawn to Work with Groups

Roselle Kurland
Robert Salmon

SUMMARY. Within the social work profession, one's world view, one's beliefs and values based on one's experiences, strongly influences one's practice and comfort with groups. This paper will examine some of the different ways of viewing the world held by practitioners and stu-dents in relation to the likelihood that they will be able to work effec-tively with groups. Such examination, and the identification of the differences among social workers that results from it has implications for both teaching and supervision in social work. These implications will be discussed and specific principles and techniques for teaching social workers, in education and in supervision, based on their world views will be described. This paper aims to enrich education for group work so that the community of social group work practitioners can grow and con-tinue to thrive. *[Article copies available for a fee from The Haworth Document Delivery Service: 1-800-HAWORTH. E-mail address: <docdelivery@haworthpress. com> Website: <http://www.HaworthPress.com> © 2006 by The Haworth Press, Inc. All rights reserved.]*

Originally published in 1999, *Journal of Teaching in Social Work,* 19(1/2), 123-137.
Reprinted with an introduction by Robert Salmon.

[Haworth co-indexing entry note]: "Education for the Group Worker's Reality: The Special Qualities and World View of Those Drawn to Work with Groups." Kurland, Roselle, and Robert Salmon. Co-published si-multaneously in *Social Work with Groups* (The Haworth Press, Inc.) Vol. 29, No. 2/3, 2006, pp. 73-89; and: *Making Joyful Noise: The Art, Science, and Soul of Group Work* (ed: Andrew Malekoff, Robert Salmon, and Dominique Moyse Steinberg) The Haworth Press, Inc., 2006, pp. 73-89. Single or multiple copies of this arti-cle are available for a fee from The Haworth Document Delivery Service [1-800-HAWORTH, 9:00 a.m. - 5:00 p.m. (EST). E-mail address: docdelivery@haworthpress.com].

73

KEYWORDS. Group work, social work education, world view

INTRODUCTION

The impetus for this article was a comment by a group work student who was reflecting on the conflict and turmoil in her group of adolescents. There was noise, disagreement and anger among the members. The student said "It was difficult and messy–but we need to stay in the mess." She was able to tolerate a very troubling situation and stay with it until there was conflict resolution.

This student referred to her work as the "mess" of ongoing efforts to work effectively with group members. Others have called it the muck, or the morass. One distinguished scholar, Donald Schon, described work of this intensity as akin to making the choice ". . . to descend to the swamp of important problems . . ." (1986, p. 3). Whatever the word or phrase chosen as the metaphor for this difficult but essential work in which the group needs to engage, it is clear that the work is neither antiseptic nor detached.

Group work students and practitioners are most likely to choose to work in the swamp of important problems. They tend to understand that the thorough exploration and resolution of conflict is often the most crucial work to be achieved by the group (Steinberg, 1993). In fact, this gritty, unpredictable, often humbling, but ultimately satisfying work, where there is an expectation that things will go wrong sometime during the process (Gitterman and Shulman, 1994), has an appeal to those who choose to practice group work. In order to do this successfully, it requires a belief in the possibility of mutual aid, patience, skill, and understanding of self and others.

Roselle Kurland and I often wondered what led students to choose this rocky road. Over time, we came to believe that the world views of group work students were crucial to their method preference. This article discusses the evolution of our thinking and offers implications for teaching as well as practice.

Robert Salmon

REFERENCES

Gitterman, A. and Shulman, L. (1994). *Mutual aid groups, vulnerable populations, and the life cycle* (2nd edition). New York: Columbia University Press.

Schon, D. (1987). *Educating the reflective practitioner*. San Francisco: Jossey Bass Publishers

Steinberg, D.M. (1987). Some findings from a study on the impact of group work education on social work with groups. *Social Work with Groups*. 16(3), 41-54.

IT'S A BIRD. IT'S A PLANE. IT'S SUPERMAN!

Consider Superman, an idealized hero from the comic books of childhood. Strong, noble, able to resolve all conflicts, Superman always was clear in setting and enforcing positive norms of behavior. Even children could describe him and his attributes.

So, how come–for a brief moment–the citizens of Metropolis didn't know if the object flying in the sky was a bird, or a plane, or Superman? The citizens had to take a moment to process the fact that while many things fly, that shared characteristic per se did not define anything. Rather, differences had to be recognized in order to make an accurate identification. Also, the differences had to be valued so that people could attend to each flying object appropriately.

The reference to Superman provides the segue to the topic of this essay, "Education for the Group Worker's Reality . . ." Certainly we can realistically assume that all social workers and social work students share common values, purposes, and characteristics. After all, they have chosen social work as their profession and the commonalities that resulted in that choice need to be recognized, identified, and appreciated.

But there are also important differences among social workers, differences in their world views[1] and in the ways in which they prioritize the many values and purposes that shape the social work profession. It is ironic that today, at a time when our profession is placing great emphasis on cultural, racial and even sexual diversity and difference, we are simultaneously ignoring the diversity of world views among ourselves.

The differences in our values, purposes, and views of the world are often reflected in the unit of service with which we prefer to work, be it group, individual, or community. Even at a time when most social workers have been educated in schools of social work whose curricula have offered generic practice courses, most social workers have a method of practice which they prefer and with which they are most comfortable.

Those preferences are rooted in the personal histories and experiences that shaped their world views and the consequent values and purposes they hold most dear. Though all social workers may subscribe to common professional values and purposes, each social worker may prioritize and operationalize a highly personal constellation of core values and purposes that are most important to him/herself. Those who prefer community organization, for example, may have entered social work out of a commitment to work toward social justice, while those who prefer to work with individuals may value individual self-determination above all (Kaiser, 1996). For group workers, Anderson's comments (1997) are germane. "In forming groups and in facilitating them, it is most helpful to discover from others their *own world views*. These include their beliefs regarding locus of control [beliefs regarding the consequences of behavior] and locus of responsibility [beliefs about the causes of behavior] and how these beliefs are applied to their interpretation of their own and others' behavior" (p. 60).

This paper will discuss and examine the world view, belief systems, and special qualities, attributes, and inclinations that characterize those social workers and social work students for whom group work is the method of choice. Implications for social work education and supervision will be suggested.

EXPOSITION

Constructivist thinking suggests that " . . . there are many truths and there are many ways of knowing. Each discovery contributes to our knowledge, and each way of knowing deepens our understanding and adds another dimension to our view of the world" (Hartman, 1990, p. 3). Group workers clearly have their own way of knowing and often a different world view from other social workers. They are ". . . a special breed of social worker with different roots, traditions, and heroes" (Middleman, 1992, p. 25).

In his book, *Educating the Reflective Practitioner*, Donald Schon (1986) talked about difference in the nature of professionals:

> In the varied topography of professional practice, there is a high, hard ground overlooking a swamp. On the high ground, manageable problems lend themselves to solution through the application of research-based theory and technique. In the swampy lowland, messy, confusing problems defy technical solution. The irony of this situation is that the problems of the high ground tend to be relatively unimportant to individuals or society at large, however great their technical interest may be, while in the swamp lie the

problems of greatest human concern. The practitioner must choose. Shall they remain on high ground where they can solve relatively unimportant problems according to prevailing standards of rigor, or shall they descend to the swamp of important problems . . . (p. 3)

Group workers tend to be among those who choose to deal with the swamp of important problems. This difference was first reflected in the historical roots of the method and prevails today.

Historically, group work was tied to early progressive education, recreation and camping, the work of the settlement houses and Jewish Centers. Group workers embraced John Dewey's educational and philosophical approach and used program activities of all kinds as the means to achieve group goals. Activities were used for enjoyment as well as to solve problems.

As Toseland and Rivas (1995, p. 48) describe, "The focus on innovative techniques and social change led to action. Compared to caseworkers, who relied on insight development from psychodynamic approaches and the provision of concrete resources, group workers relied on program activities to spur members to action." Exemplary of the difference, group workers preferred to say members rather than clients (Bowman, 1935, as quoted in Toseland and Rivas, p. 49) and clearly emphasized members' strengths rather than their weaknesses.

Tracing the history of group work within the profession, Middleman (1992) said:

> . . . Group workers were different, often were thought of as unprofessional by the caseworkers. They worked at night, even venturing into the "bad" neighborhoods, were out of the office more than behind the desk, and went camping with their group members. They were women who didn't wear hats and men in plaid shirts without suitcoats and neckties. They were workers who enjoyed having a meal or a party with their people, who used activities like singing and dancing, who weren't neutral but shared their beliefs . . . They were workers whose work may have appeared chaotic and not so controlled, who encouraged the community to vote and become active in political and current affairs, for they were concerned with action and social issues. (p. 26)

But, professional social work became defined as casework (Wenocur and Reisch, 1989, p. 225), and it was only in 1935 that group work became linked formally with social work at the National Conference of Social Work. Even then, it was reported that in 1936 ". . . the California Conference of Social Work seriously questioned whether group workers were social workers. Faculty members of the School of Social Administration of the University of Chicago minced no words in their exclusion of any study of an activity remotely connected with recreation" (Wilson, 1976).

In a plenary paper delivered at the 16th Annual Symposium on Social Work with Groups, Wood and Middleman (1996) discussed constructivism and the theme that how one views the world is strongly influenced by one's experiences in that world. Each person's reality is different. This idea also can be applied to the way we view the place of group work within the social work profession. Group work was forced to struggle for legitimacy and recognition. That experience helped our method survive. It helped us develop elegant ways of involving our clients in shared decision-making that strengthened our practice. It helped us, according to our interpretation of reality, to develop passion and commitment, skill in dealing with conflict, a love of action, humor in adversity, and a tolerance for tumult that is effective for practice today. The history of group work has been an important factor in producing a world view that is different from the world views of many other social workers with other method orientations.

Over the years, certain attitudes and values seem to characterize social workers and social work students who are drawn to group work practice and to be intrinsic to their world view. They are also elements that are crucial in the conceptual and emotional foundation of group work practice today.

Group workers believe in and emphasize the strengths of the group members.

Belief in the strengths of people is at the heart of group work practice. In fact, the very act of forming a group is a statement of belief in the strengths of those who are to become group members, a statement of belief that each person who is asked to join a group has something to offer and to give to the other members as well as to receive from them. This is in sharp contrast to a pathology perspective that views a person's illness, weaknesses, and problems as central.

Group workers see the client as a social being in interaction with others rather than as an individual puzzle to be solved or fixed. In fact, group workers are often concerned about changing systems and not just persons (Breton, 1989). They emphasize participatory democracy, social justice, and the duties and obligations owed others (Lewis, 1989). They concentrate on assessing need and resources rather than making a diagnosis.

Last year, a student in one of the author's group work classes was placed in an alternative junior high school for teens identified as "behaviorally disturbed." Their classroom teacher insisted on attending the group she led and, during the course of the group meetings, would often whisper to this student to be stricter and keep the members more firmly "in control." In fact, "control" seemed to be a word this teacher used and acted upon continuously, so much so that the student described herself as feeling intimidated, uptight, unnatural, and more of a disciplinarian in the group than she thought she needed to be. Fortunately, a heavy winter snow fall necessitated the student's leading the group one day without the teacher present. At this meeting, she resolved to relinquish the heavy-handed control she had felt forced to adopt. Much to her delight, when a group member would misbehave, another member would tell him, "Hey, cut it out. She trusts us." The student's decision to relinquish control and to trust in the strengths of the group members proved transformational in the life of the group and proved to the student that when treated with respect and high expectations the members responded positively and demonstrated strengths previously hidden. Eventually, this student was able to communicate this to her teacher/co-leader as well as to other teachers and staff at the school who, seeing the way the members responded in the group that she led, began coming to her for advice about groups they were leading or wanted to form.

Similar stories can certainly be told about other students who, when they arrive at their field work agencies with enthusiasm and many ideas for potential groups, are discouraged by staff at the agency and told that the clients won't (come to a group, be willing to try a new activity, etc.) or can't (participate in group discussion, interact with one another, sit still for very long, etc.) If the student is persistent and does not lose hope or enthusiasm, more often than not they (and the staff!) discover that the clients will and can and do! Such is the power of believing in client strengths and of acting upon that belief!

Group workers believe in mutual aid and do not feel the need to be in full control of the interchange among group members.

Mutual aid is at the heart of group work practice. It refers to members helping one another as they think things through. It relies on spontaneous communication and interaction among group members. Mutual aid has little room to develop when group members interact primarily with the worker while their co-members watch and listen. Thus, mutual aid relies on the exchange of strengths among group members. It has little room to develop when it is the practitioner who is regarded as the principal helper in the group (Steinberg, 1997).

Mutual aid means that many voices contribute to the helping process in the group and there is mutual interdependence. Often, the worker is not in control and the process may sometimes seem chaotic to the outsider. The group practitioner realizes and even relishes the idea that in the life of the group there are important actors other than him/herself. It takes a particular kind of person to find this appealing, to respond favorably to the idea of the sharing of power, control, and decision making that characterizes mutual aid in the group.

Group workers find the unpredictability of a group, the fact that one never quite knows what will take place in a group meeting, exciting and stimulating rather than threatening. They are comfortable with "messiness," with seeming disorder, with the many voices of a group that may make it seem chaotic at times. They accept fallibility as inevitable, a corollary to sharing control.

Those who are drawn to group work tend to believe that true sharing and interchange will often be "noisy." Hence, they do not think they have failed or blame themselves when the many voices of the group are being expressed with intensity. Those who are new to group work practice may, at first, believe that they should take responsibility on their shoulders alone for all that takes place in the group. But they quickly learn that they cannot be, do not have to be, and even do not want to be "in control" of all that takes place in the group. Throwing things back to the group, making observations to the group about what s/he sees taking place rather than solving problems for the group quickly becomes the group worker's way of work. In fact, students of group work are relieved, increasingly comfortable, and find group work to be fun and exciting when they realize they do not need or want to have all the answers, that they can be honest with the group about things that they see.

The idea of expecting things to go wrong in the group is a crucial one (Gitterman and Shulman, 1994). Group workers know that neither the group nor the worker will achieve perfection from the beginning. They realize that there will be ebbs and flows, success and regression. They are comfortable with that and do not blame themselves or see it as their failure when the group enters a difficult phase. The patience and skill needed to endure and flourish in this kind of interchange requires special characteristics in the practitioner. As one group work student exclaimed, "We need to stay in the 'mess.'"

Group workers value difference. They see conflict as a natural and expectable element of group life.

Because they are comfortable with the "mess" and "noise" of a group, group workers understand the value and importance of conflict and the expression of difference in the group. They do not rush to quash conflict or to resolve it superficially or prematurely so the group can move on. They realize that the exploration and resolution of conflict the real work of the group (see Steinberg, 1993). They do not overreact to conflict, nor are they afraid of it.

An example of this was expressed recently in a group work class. A student whose internship was at a day treatment program for the mentally ill described what she thought was a wonderful group session in which disagreement among members was being expressed. "I didn't even realize it, but I guess it must have gotten loud," she said. "Because all of a sudden one of the workers at the agency came into the room and wanted to know if everything was alright. I think she was worried that things had gotten out of control, but what was taking place was great. There was nothing to be worried about." The student understood, implicitly, that it was not her function to try to save the group from its conflict by doing its work for it. Workers need to let the process continue rather than bringing it to closure quickly and prematurely (Henry, 1992, p. 151). It that occurs, the conflict, unresolved, will only emerge later. The ability to appreciate and accept difference and conflict, to be comfortable with them, reflects the world view of those who are drawn to work with groups.

Group workers appreciate the commonalities of the human experience and are able to see those commonalities even in seemingly different situations. It is that vision of commonalities that enables them to practice group work rather than casework in a group.

The practice of group work requires that workers be able to see the opportunity for all in the group that is presented by the issues and questions raised by one of the group's members (Kurland and Salmon, 1993). Thus, the worker needs to be able to "think group" (Middleman and Wood, 1990, p. 97) and help the group members not merely sit back and almost antiseptically offer advice to the group member who is raising an issue. Group members need to be helped to look at their own experiences and situations. Even if they have not had the exact experience or faced exactly the same issue that is being raised by one group member, all the members have experiences that are relevant. The advice that group members ultimately offer needs to be rooted in the examination of their own experiences that one member's issues provide the opportunity for all in the group to do.

Thus, group work is very different from casework in a group, different from a round robin approach in which members take turns one-by-one, different from what Hartford (1978, p. 25) called the "aggregational therapy of individuals." The practice of group work, therefore, requires an ability to conceptualize on the part of the worker, a broad vision that enables him/her to see, appreciate, draw upon, and link what is common in what may appear at first to be unique.

Group workers do not see themselves as neutral observers. They believe that using themselves actively in the group and "lending a vision" (Schwartz, 1971) can be of great value and they are comfortable doing so.

Social workers who work with groups tend to be persons who prefer to take an active rather than a passive stance in/with a group. They express their points of view and professional knowledge in the group and challenge group members' thinking. With judgment, they artfully use their "understanding and knowledge to express a point of view without imposing that view on the group and its members, in such a way that members feel free to question, to challenge, to wonder, to disagree (or agree) and thereby further define their own beliefs and points of view" (Kurland and Malekoff, 1996).

Group workers model and provide active support and guidance in solving immediate problems. They tend to not be comfortable functioning as a tabula rasa, " . . . a symbolic figure who passively invites perceptions of him/herself to be guided by the group members' individual and collective unconscious needs . . ." and who encourages " . . . intensive transference relationships both positive and negative, regressive catharsis, free association, and deep exploration of members' histories" (Garland, 1986, p. 19).

Instead, group workers are persons who tend to be comfortable sharing of themselves, their successes, uncertainties, and even mistakes, with a group. They are courageous. When their own experiences, positive and/or negative, might be helpful to the learning of group members, they do not hesitate to share them with the group. Important here is that their sharing of experiences is aimed toward meeting the needs of the group members rather than their own needs (to be accepted or liked, for example).

Group workers are comfortable with their own authority in/with a group.

Though students with a preference for group work practice often enter social work school with the belief that work with groups will allow them to be "one of the gang" (see Kurland and Salmon, 1993), they quickly learn that they are and need to be figures of authority in the groups with which they work. They come to understand that the way in which they use their authority differs, depending on the group's needs and stage of development. In beginnings, for example, when a group needs structure, limits, direction, and guidance to establish norms of behavior and clarify purpose, the worker needs to assert his/her authority more actively. Later, in the middle stages, as the group develops the ability to provide its own direction, the need for the worker to actively assert his/her authority lessens.

Perhaps because they were reluctant to exert authority at first, workers' early experiences in working with groups clearly demonstrate to them the need for them to do so. This results in group workers rapidly becoming increasingly comfortable exercising skills of authority. They come to see that to not provide the direction, structure and limits that a beginning group needs is to abdicate the responsibility of serving the group with the best skill available (Henry, 1992, p. 115). Comfort with authority characterizes or comes to characterize workers with groups.

Group workers are creative.

It has been said, that " . . . people trained in creative thinking and problem solving are superior in analytical thinking, in divergent thinking, and in the ability to suspend judgment and generate options" (Weissman, 1990, p. 251). The ingredients necessary for the creative process to flourish have been described as

> . . . seeing things in a new way, making connections, taking risks, being alerted to chance and to the opportunities present(ed) by

contradictions and complexities, recognizing familiar patterns in the unfamiliar so that new patterns may be formed by transforming old ones, being alert to the contingencies which may arise from such transformations. (Barron and Harrington, 1985, p. 168)

These ingredients are close to what Dewey called for in his third stage of the problem-solving process, the thorough exploration and consideration of all conceivable solutions to a problem (Morris and Pai, 1976, p. 149). The ability to learn how to be effective in the problem solving process, so essential to group workers, appears to be directly connected to creativity. Similarly, the ability to plan with thoroughness also allows the group worker to be spontaneous, when indicated. "Talented social workers must be talented improvisers. Policies and program . . . cannot completely fit the complexities or exigencies of life. Great improvisers make novel creative connections" (Weissman, 1990, p. 254)

Group workers come from a tradition where thorough exploration of an issue, and spontaneity are seen as the two inseparable sides of one coin. Group workers are persons who welcome and enjoy the many opportunities for artistry, innovation and creativity that work with groups provides.

IMPLICATIONS FOR SOCIAL WORK EDUCATION

From the 1960s on, as the Council on Social Work Education moved toward curriculum standards that required schools of social work to emphasize the generic in social work practice, the differences in the world views and value orientations among social work students have been largely ignored and swept under the rug. The commonalities of all methods and, by implication, the commonalities among all social workers were greatly emphasized. But to neglect the differences and diversity among social work students and practitioners is to overgeneralize and to deprive our profession of that which enriches us all. As David Howe (1980) commented:

About of thinking generic has caused people in the personal social services to seek out the common characteristics of those who work in the field and then announce that these shared attributes are, in fact, the real and essential characteristics of all social workers. By definition, generic qualities are wider and more encompassing than specific characteristics. But merely to say that all lions and tigers are just cats, and henceforth only cats are to be recognized, not only makes for a bad taxonomy but also might confuse those who wish to know how to catch mice or go big game hunting. (p. 318)

It is, perhaps, incongruous that as social workers we know and appreciate the value of diversity and difference in the groups with which we work, and the important role they play in providing stimulation, yet we seem to have forgotten their importance to our profession. Increasingly, as research has shown (see Goldberg and Lamont, 1992; Birnbaum and Auerbach, 1994), social work students in their education are less exposed to the literature, roots, traditions and practice of group work. As a result, those students whose value orientations and world views may predispose them toward the group work method, always a minority within social work, may come to question whether they belong and/or have a place in social work.

This was clearly illustrated recently at the Hunter College School of Social Work, where the authors teach, a School that has maintained a method-specific curriculum. The first year that a new Foundations course was added for first-year students, courses in each method did not begin immediately but instead started five weeks into the semester. When the group work classes met for the first time that year, one student expressed the view of many in group work when she loudly stated at the end of the first class session, "Whew, it's a relief to have this class. I was beginning to wonder whether social work was for me." Another student quickly added, "I feel so alone in the Foundations course. Here there's support and people who think more like I do." A third student followed, "This class shouldn't start later than the others. Next year, start it right at the beginning."

To support and strengthen the world view and values of those who are drawn to the practice of group work, social work educators need to do a number of things.

First, we need to continue to help our students and supervisees appreciate the commonalities in the values that provide social work's foundations. Simultaneously, we need to help them recognize, appreciate and even celebrate the differences in world views and values that lead them to prefer a specific social work method (Kaiser, 1996). We need to help students identify and prioritize the values that are central to them and that motivated their choice of social work as a profession. We need to acknowledge and recognize that these values and the ways in which individual students prioritize them will differ for different students.

Second, as teachers of social work we need to identify our own world views, central values and priorities, to admit that we have them rather than to ignore that fact by continuing to say we ascribe to all values equally. Helpful in defining and differentiating our own value preferences is a question we might ask ourselves: When we work with students, what is it that they report doing that we find really exciting? For the authors of this paper, the importance we place on client strengths was underscored when we asked ourselves that question, for we found that what excites us, above all, is when students are successful in helping clients to succeed when others (e.g., colleagues, other staff, supervisors, etc.) thought they could or would not.

Third, we need to help students find sub-communities within social work that will nurture and help them further develop their vision of and passion for social work. The support and strength that one gains from finding others who share important commonalities, so central to group work practice, applies to our students and supervisees as well.

In an earlier paper (Salmon, Getzel and Kurland, 1991), the authors discussed the learning styles of four types of learners who had different levels of skill in and knowledge about group work. One, characterized as the "Thinker," knew group work literature and theory but had limited skills and experience. The "Natural" had considerable experience with groups, significant skill, and an aversion to the analysis and conceptualization of his/her practice. The "Neophyte" had relatively little of both knowledge and skill, and the "Star" is a student blessed with a modest but well integrated level of both. Differential methods of teaching group work to these different kinds of learners were presented so that teachers of group work could match their expectations for learning with the individual needs and evolving styles of their students.

Now, a fourth recommendation is that we add to this typology the dimension of values and world view as a teaching consideration. Doing so would strengthen our teaching. Some students, for example, who are learning about groups may find it difficult to support mutual aid. They may need special help to see client strengths and/or to not overly control the group. Others may need help to become comfortable with their role of authority. Still others may need help to be more accepting of the "noise" and "mess" of the group and of their own fallibility.

CONCLUSION

Students enter graduate school with a world view that has shaped their values and belief system. They enter the educational process with a vision of who they are, and what they would like to do and become. Students who are drawn to group work practice share some unique views, values, qualities and attributes. These need to be recognized and taken into account in social work teaching. The essence of some of these special qualities were captured by Middleman (1992) in an Association for the Advancement of Social Work With Groups (AASWG) plenary address:

> Social Work with Groups . . . is a mentality–a perspective, a way of looking at the world that is learned when one studies basic group theory and practice. It takes time and practice to learn to focus on several and their human context before zeroing in on the particular one, to observe differently–look at the broad picture, see what's happening and not happening, think purpose before content, strengths of clients and not simply the problems, and to be eager to give your power away to others without feeling uncomfortable. (p. 35)

Group work persists today and may be in the first stages of a renaissance. The use of groups is growing. Even the CSWE has recognized the value of groups and has moved, albeit with excruciating and exasperating slowness, to bring educational content in the group work method back into the social work curriculum. The few schools that continue group work specializations have a consistent demand for admission. The number of group work elective courses apparently has expanded in other schools. Many students and applicants want to learn about groups. Recognizing the unique world views and values of those drawn to group work practice may enable us to enrich and strengthen our group work teaching.

NOTE

1. World view has become increasingly important as an intrinsic part of the conceptual frame of reference of social workers. It fits into constructionist thinking. "According to constructionists, meanings arise in particular settings or traditions. The communities and cultures of which we are members determine our ways of seeing the

world" (Gergen, p. 128). Furthermore, the constructionist point of view clearly indicates that " . . . individual and interpersonal ways of making meaning are situated in larger contexts and come from the social domains of which we are a part" (Dean, p. 142). Middleman and Rhodes (1985) elaborated on this. "World views have been discussed in different disciplines under diverse labels, for example, paradigms, models, structures of reasoning, epistemologies. They have been called patterns of thought (Pribram, 1949) and the 'pattern which connects–the metapattern or pattern of patterns' " (Bateson, 1979, p. 48). Middleman and Rhodes emphasized the use and importance of world view in their formulation. They think of it as " . . . a meta-view or frame of reference or metaphor or belief system; this world view influences our beliefs about 'being in the universe,' and leads to 'the models' we pose" (p. 49).

REFERENCES

Anderson, J. (1997). *Social Work with Groups: A Process Model*. New York: Longman.

Barron, F. and Harrington, D. (1985). Creativity. In A. Kuper and J. Kuper (Eds.). *The Social Science Encyclopedia* (pp. 167-169). London: Routledge and Kegan Paul.

Bateson, G. (1979). *Mind and Nature: A Necessary Unity*. New York: Elsevier-Dutton.

Birnbaum, M.L. and Auerbach, C. (1994). Group work in graduate social work education: The practice of neglect. *Journal of Social Work Education*, 30(3), 325-335.

Bowman, L. (1935). Dictatorship, democracy and group work in America. In *Proceedings of the National Conference of Social Work* (p. 382). Chicago: University of Chicago Press.

Breton, M. (1989, October). Learning from social group work traditions. *Proceedings of the Eleventh Annual Symposium on Social Work with Groups*. Montreal, Canada.

Dean, R. Grossman. (1993). Constructivism: An approach to clinical practice. *Smith College Studies in Social Work, 63* (2), March, pp. 127-146.

Garland, J. (1986). The relationship between social group work and group therapy: Can a group therapist be a social group worker, too? In M. Parnes, (ed.), *Innovations in Social Group Work: Feedback from Practice to Theory*. New York: The Haworth Press, Inc., pp. 17-28.

Gergen, K. (1985). The social constructionist movement in modern psychology. *American Psychologist, 40* (3), pp. 266-275.

Gitterman, A. and Shulman, L. (1994). *Mutual Aid Groups, Vulnerable Populations, and the Life Cycle*, second edition. New York: Columbia University Press.

Goldberg, T. and Lamont, A. (1992). The impact of a generic curriculum on the practice of graduates: Does group work persist? *Social Work with Groups*, 15 (2/3), 145-156.

Hartford, M. (1971). *Group in Social Work*. New York: Columbia University Press.

Hartman, A. (1990). Many Ways of Knowing. *Social Work*, 35(1), Editorial, pp. 3-4.

Henry, S. (1992). *Group Skills–A Four Dimensional Approach*, second edition. Pacific Grove, CA: Brooks/Cole Publishing Company.

Howe, D. (1980). Inflated states and empty theories in social work. *The British Journal of Social Work,* 10 (3), pp. 317-340.

Kaiser, M. (1996). Some uncommon frameworks of social work practice. Unpublished paper, Hunter College School of Social Work.

Kurland, R. and Malekoff, A. (1996). Editorial, *Social Work with Groups, 19* (3/4).

Kurland, R. and Salmon, R. (1993). Group work vs. casework in a group: Implications for teaching and practice. *Groupwork,* 6 (1), pp. 5-16, also in *Social Work with Groups,* 15 (4), (1992).

Kurland, R. and Salmon, R. (1993). Not just one of the gang: Group workers and their roles as an authority. *Social Work with Groups,* 16 (1/2), pp. 153-169.

Lewis, H. (1989). Transcript from videotaped panel, Hunter College School of Social Work. (October 3).

Middleman, R. and Rhodes, G. (1985). *Competent Supervision: Making Imaginative Judgments.* Englewood Cliffs, New Jersey: Prentice Hall.

Middleman, R. (1992). Group work and the Heimlich Maneuver: Unchoking social work education. In D. Fike & B. Rittner, (Eds.) *Working from Strengths: The Essence of Group Work.* Miami, Florida: Center for Group Work Studies, pp. 16-39.

Middleman, R. and Wood, G. (1990). *Skills for Direct Practice in Social Work.* New York: Columbia University Press.

Morris, V.C. and Pai, Y. (1976). *Philosophy and The American School,* second edition. Boston, MA: Houghton Mifflin Company.

Pribam, K. (1949). *Conflicting Patterns of Thought.* Washington, DC: Public Affairs Press.

Salmon, R., Getzel, G., and Kurland, R. (1991). The neophyte, the natural, the thinker and the star. *Journal of Teaching in Social Work,* 5 (1), 65-80.

Schon, D. (1987). *Educating The Reflective Practitioner.* San Francisco: Jossey Bass Publishers.

Schwartz, W. (1971). On the use of groups in social work practice. In W. Schwartz and S. Zalba, (Eds.). *The Practice of Group Work.* New York: Columbia University Press.

Schwartz, W. (1961). The social worker in the group. *The Social Welfare Forum, Proceedings of the National Conference on Social Welfare.* New York: Columbia University Press.

Steinberg, D. (1997). *The Mutual Aid Approach to Working with Groups: Helping People Help Each Other.* New Jersey: Jason Aronson, Inc.

Steinberg, D. (1993). Some findings from a study on the impact of group work education on social work with groups. *Social Work with Groups.* 16 (3), 41-54.

Toseland, R. and Rivas, R. (1995). *An Introduction to Group Work Practice,* second edition. Boston, MA: Allyn and Bacon.

Weissman, H. (1990). *Serious Play: Creativity and Innovation in Social Work.* Silver Spring, MD: National Association of Social Workers.

Wenocur, S. and Reisch, M. (1989). *From Charity to Enterprise: The Development of Social Work in a Market Economy.* Urbana: University of Illinois Press.

Wilson, G. (1976). From practice to theory: A personalized history. In R. Roberts & H. Northen, (Eds.). *Theories of Social Work with Groups.* New York: Columbia University Press.

Wood, G. and Middleman, R.(1996). Constructivism, power, and social work with groups. In J. Parry, (Ed.). *From Prevention to Wellness Through Group Work.* New York: The Haworth Press, Inc.

Organizational Insight and the Education of Advanced Group Work Practitioners

Harriet Goodman

SUMMARY. This article is the second piece about a group work course designed for advanced work-study students who are not in field placement. It discusses how group workers can use organizational analysis to improve group work practice in agencies with both social conflict and social transition functions. Practice examples illustrate how students promote group work principles in settings where the method has historically had limited currency. *[Article copies available for a fee from The Haworth Document Delivery Service: 1-800-HAWORTH. E-mail address: <docdelivery@haworthpress.com> Website: <http://www.HaworthPress.com> © 2006 by The Haworth Press, Inc. All rights reserved.]*

KEYWORDS. Group work education, group work practice, organizational analysis

INTRODUCTION

Since the 1970s concerns about the erosion of social group work practice have continued to vex professionals committed to the method (Tropp, 1978). The literature describes the deterioration in group work

The author wishes to thank the One-Year Residency Group Work Class of January 2006 for their invaluable contributions to this article.

[Haworth co-indexing entry note]: "Organizational Insight and the Education of Advanced Group Work Practitioners." Goodman, Harriet. Co-published simultaneously in *Social Work with Groups* (The Haworth Press, Inc.) Vol. 29, No. 2/3, 2006, pp. 91-104; and: *Making Joyful Noise: The Art, Science, and Soul of Group Work* (ed: Andrew Malekoff, Robert Salmon, and Dominique Moyse Steinberg) The Haworth Press, Inc., 2006, pp. 91-104. Single or multiple copies of this article are available for a fee from The Haworth Document Delivery Service [1-800-HAWORTH, 9:00 a.m. - 5:00 p.m. (EST). E-mail address: docdelivery@haworthpress.com].

doi:10.1300/J009v29n02_07

practice, supervision and education (Kurland and Salmon, 2002; Middleman, 1990; Newman, 2000; Tropp, 1978). However, few authors use structural analysis to consider how the broader organizational context of contemporary social work practice influences what group work practice models a particular venue would most embrace or how workers can adapt practice to changes in the social service environment (Bitel, 2005; Doel and Sawdon, 1999; Garland, 1992). Although Kurland's Model for Group Work Planning (Northen and Kurland, 2001) invites workers to consider the agency context, group workers focus on the micro aspects of pre-group planning, such as composition, purpose, need, structure and content.

This article draws on the experiences of students in an advanced social group work class that uses a typology of agency purpose based on Glasser and Garvin's (1979) Organizational Model, which serves as a guide to understand the relationship between organization function and group programs in their agencies. This paper builds on a previous article about the same advanced group work class. The previous article identifies contemporary problems in social group work and describes how group practitioners routinely find solutions to problems of practice (Goodman and Munoz, 2004). The current article uses examples from students' class assignments to demonstrate how group practice can thrive when workers analyze the purpose and dynamic needs of the agency where they are employed. It concludes with a discussion of how an analytic approach to organizational purpose and the changing context of practice can help these workers promote groups that are consistent with agency purpose and social group work principles.

THE DECLINE OF GROUP WORK PRACTICE AND THEORY

In 1978 Emmanuel Tropp identified conditions contributing to the deterioration of social group work practice. He documented the increase of generic methods education that began in 1965, a period during which enrollment in graduate social work schools was increasing. Micromethods practice that incorporated casework and group work into a single generic practice course decreased instruction in the individual methods. Tropp began what became a refrain in successive decades: when casework and group work are taught as generalist practice, social group work practice suffers. Group work specialization decreased, and the development of group work theory diminished. Ultimately, these trends reinforced each other, and the core roots of social group work gradually began to wear away (Tropp, 1978).

By the 1990s group work luminaries were expressing alarm about the state of social group work. The Annual Symposium on Social Work with Groups became the venue for a series of impassioned plenary addresses that called upon Symposium attendees to preserve the historical standards of social work with groups (Kurland, 2003; Kurland and Salmon, 1992, 2002; Middleman, 1990). Because the audience for these addresses was primarily people already committed to social group work, however, they had limited influence beyond the converted.

At the same time, group workers studied problems in social group work education. Strozier (1997) analyzed teaching methods from syllabi gathered from the AASWG collection of graduate group work courses. The courses relied heavily on experiential learning and did not reflect consensus regarding texts, content or integration of field in the classroom. The work of Birnbaum with Auerbach (1994) and Wayne (2000) focused more on the educators themselves. Social work educators assigned themselves high ratings in teaching practice; at the same time they were unable to identify important group work concepts. These researchers view the problem through an educational lens and promote curriculum standards that include group work content (Birnbaum and Auerbach, 1994; Birnbaum and Wayne, 2000).

Evidently, additional group work content in social work education would result in better direct group practice (Hines, 2005). Steinberg (1993), who explored the differences between social workers who received and did not receive specialized group work education, found that practitioners with more than two semesters of graduate group education promoted mutual aid, were more comfortable with conflict, exercised less control and titrated "use of self" in a manner consistent with the stage of the group (Steinberg, 1993).

Ironically, at the same time that education in social group work diminished, the need for highly skilled, uniquely educated social group workers expanded (Garland, 1992). As a result, other professional and paraprofessional groups have moved into the breech and assumed roles that have been historically the purview of social group workers. This, along with the current penchant for evidence-based practices that can easily be replicated by people with limited or no human services training (Tanenbaum, 2005), has led to the proliferation of curricula that unschooled group leaders can follow to conduct groups with any number of populations (Kurland and Malekoff, 1998). In the areas of mental health, substance abuse, parenting skills, or anger management, for example, evidence-based practices include a number of groups based on curricula, some of which Kurland and Malekoff (1998) would describe as "curriculum driven," while others offer the group worker more latitude (Goodman, 2002).

Another consequence of the contraction of group work education in social work graduate programs is the isolation that newly graduated group workers experience and the lack of administrative support to propose and conduct appropriate group services. Although some report tension between their low status as new employees and the desire of other workers to exploit their expert knowledge about group practice (Newman, 1999), others find ways to bring their group work expertise to both clients and the agencies in which they work (Goodman and Munoz, 2004) or encourage professional development groups to benefit workers and promote an optimistic view of the future of social group work (Bergart and Simon, 2005).

THE ADVANCED GROUP WORK PRACTICE COURSE

The need for an advanced group work class to teach work-study students who were no longer under the protection of their group work field assignment became evident when the author was assigned the course. Because of a scheduling fluke, all members of the first class were one-year residency students who would graduate within four months. This cohort rejected the historic content of the course because it was irrelevant in their current circumstances. The standard course outline was identical to a second section, where all of the students were in their second year of course work and field work placement. Unlike the Two-Year students, the work-study students did not need to hone practice skills; they needed skills to bridge the gulf between what they had learned in two intensive semesters of social group work study and their current employment as agency-based group workers and supervisors.

Thus, with the encouragement and support of Professor Kurland, the course outline was revised. Through an inductive process that included a critical incident assignment to identify problems that group work employees experience in their jobs, the focus of the course became how workers were promoting or could promote social group work within the constraints of their organizations. Additional content about theories of group work practice expanded the practice palate for these student-workers. At the time of writing, four cohorts of students have enrolled in this special section, and the course has integrated student input over time.

THE CHALLENGE AT HAND

The first paper that described this course focused on specific problems that students identified and the solutions they developed *in situ*. Their problems mirrored those described in the social group work literature (Goodman and Munoz, 2004). In virtually all settings where they were employed, they confronted the lack of group work specialists, particularly among supervisory or administrative staff. At the same time, their agencies pressured them to increase group services. Based on examples from more than seventy enrolled in the advanced course over four years, it is clear that agencies are experiencing intense pressure to produce group services either to generate income or because of perceived demands for efficiency.

Flowing from increased demand and limited group work expertise and leadership, the students had insufficient time to plan for groups. Another result of the combination of diminished resources and increased demand for groups is the proliferation "curriculum driven" groups (Kurland and Malekoff, 1998). In some instances these problems converge so that inexperienced supervisors will provide a worker a curriculum without allocating time to prepare for the group, evaluate the appropriateness of the sessions for the members, consult with a coleader or make any adaptations or appropriate elements of the method that might be useful.

An additional problem that develops from economic or service target pressure for group services is the loss of centrality of group purpose (Kurland and Salmon, 1998). The ripple effect is apparent when members do not share any perceived need; workers are not permitted pregroup contact with members, and activity is rejected as a powerful group work tool even with populations for whom verbal expression is not available. A particularly egregious situation occurs when the purpose of the group is clearly the need for a group assignment for a student intern.

The first article about this course described in detail techniques that advanced group workers use to address these problems through interactions with colleagues, supervisors, and in the group itself. All student cohorts advocated for valued practice principles. They took direct action as informal "internal group work experts" by providing readings or advice. Through a technique labeled "collaborative learning" they used informal but purposeful opportunities to transmit knowledge about group work. A particularly imaginative example occurred when a student used the staff lunch table to spread out his group work planning materials and waited for the inevitable questions to arise from his co-workers. "Creative hanging out" was a strategy that enabled workers to identify unmet needs that they could capitalize on to develop groups to meet client needs.

Attenuated planning or "planning in place" was another strategy where employees would explicitly devote the first sessions of the group to planning with members. This technique was useful with all group structures: open-ended, closed, short-term, long-term, or single session groups.

Advanced group workers routinely altered curricula to suit the needs of their clients through "curricular adaptation." When curricular examples were not appropriate to the racial, cultural, or other member characteristics, they substituted examples that resonated with members. In addition, they inserted material that promoted mutual aid and shifted authority to the members, even with didactic curricula. Some of these activities took place within the confines of worker-group interactions. In other cases, workers made changes with the sanction of their agencies.

THE ORGANIZATIONAL MODEL
OF GROUP WORK PRACTICE

Although the spirited actions of individual group workers had powerful effects, they occurred without explicit analysis of the agency context and ever-changing external events that influenced the organization. In general, external events or agency purpose were viewed as impediments and not neutral boundaries that determine the nature of practice. The student-employees applied skills based on a commitment to micro practice principles; they did not address the subtleties of function in the particular agency in which they were employed.

However, Bitel (2005) underscores the importance of the agency context in her comprehensive review of the group work literature. She states that more than any other method, social group work's origins are imbedded in agency practice, and a worker's ability to negotiate informal agency structure affects the implementation of group programs (Brandler and Roman, 2005). Group work practice occurs within formal organizations and workers act must differentially based on the organization in which they work (Bitel, 2005).

Doel and Sawdon (1995, 1999) have attempted to enrich group work practice in England using an organizational perspective. They introduced intensive educational interventions within agencies and approached the development of group work programs from the perspective of the agency's systemic needs. They explain their "essentialist" model of group work through the metaphor of a house. All houses require certain structural components such as a roof, walls, doors, and windows. At the same time houses are very diverse; some features are essential and others are conditional. The specific characteristics of the house, therefore, must be developed within a context of those conditions. Similarly, group work practices must develop based on the way in which agencies interact with the wider world, particularly the specific functions for which they are established (Doel and Sawdon, 1999).

As the advanced group work practice course evolved, we directed students' attention to the organizations in which they were working. Presentation of organizational and sociological theories broadened their analytic capacities. This conceptual approach was an effort to contextualize the concrete practice problems that students wrote about in their "critical incident" assignments. A particularly useful theory was Glasser and Garvin's (1976) development of Vinter's preventive and rehabilitative approach that locates the worker's role relative to organizational and environmental conditions. Although the environmental context is dynamic and continually changing (Garvin, 1986), the Organizational Model lays out functional types that students can use as a scaffold for analytic purposes.

Glasser and Garvin propose that social agencies have two basic functions: they either (1) address social conflict or (2) help people with social transitions. Within these overarching functional types clients have different levels of motivation to participate in groups and attend for different reasons. Within the organizational category of social conflict, some agencies are given legal authority to limit deviant behavior. Services are not voluntary, and the central goal of the agency is to decrease sanctioned behaviors (Glasser and Garvin, 1976). Social conflict organizations can also have a re-socialization function, which emphasizes development of new values, knowledge or skills. There may be pressures for participation, but they would fall into the category that Rooney (1994, 2004) labels "involuntary" in contrast to "mandated," where the agency has direct or conferred legal authority for client participation in a group.

Student-workers in this class were frequently employed in social conflict settings where the client participation is either mandated or involuntary, including community and residential drug treatment programs, alternative to detention programs, homeless services, residential services for youth, schools, and certain types of child welfare services. Students expressed discomfort in acting as agents of social control or in leading groups where clients' participation was not voluntary (Rooney, 1994). Because the culture of social group work, which developed from democratic principles, assumes voluntary participation. As a result, they often labeled clients as "resistant" and felt alien within the organization. However, by locating their work within the wider purpose of the agency, the student employees were able to identify the non-negotiable aspects of the agency's mission. At the same time, they separated out areas where they had discretion in their practice and introduced changes that promoted superior group work practice. The group worker who remains informed about mandates within their agency and external forces that may alter those mandates can seize opportunities that as they arise (Rooney, 1994).

PRACTICE EXAMPLES

One student provided an example of involuntary re-socialization groups in a women's homeless shelter. Her critical incident was important because she made significant adaptations when changes in the external environment occurred:

> The setting is a homeless shelter for women. The women were mandated to attend a group or they would lose privileges. When we started, the women were all waiting for *Section Eight* housing, and the purpose of this group was to help them learn how to keep an apartment on their own (re-socialization). We had few real group workers leading these groups, and they were pretty didactic, but we tried to give members real-life examples so it would mean something to them if they ever did get a place of their own. Then the *Section Eight* program dried up, and the purpose of the group dried up too. The women were still required to attend groups, however, so I met with the three workers, and we talked about what to do. This was where my group work classes came in, because I knew about group purpose. It became clear to me that the groups could help the women learn to become advocates for themselves.

It worked out great. The other group leaders agreed to the plan. We even met with the Commissioner and our members have been going to other shelters to tell them what was happening.

This example is notable for several reasons. Although participation in the groups was involuntary in exchange for maintaining residence in the shelter, the worker identified true-to-life situations the women might actually confront. Rooney (1994) has long promoted this approach as a way of reducing "reactance," or the normal reaction people have when they lose valued freedoms (Nezlek and Brehm, 1975). He rejects the label "resistant" in these settings as a means of normalizing the predictable anger or withdrawal when people feel pressured or coerced (Rooney, 2004). In addition, this worker's opportunistic strategy in the face of a changing environment had superb results.

The second functional type of organization helps people who are making life transitions. These agencies can address situations in which clients are having difficulties with social functioning. Another type of social transition agency serves people who are moving from one developmental stage to another. Although adults may attend these groups voluntarily, children may be required to participate in group programs. Nonetheless, these organizations tend to have more flexible rules and decision making is more democratic than in social control organizations (Glasser and Garvin, 1976).

A student working in a sub-acute rehabilitation nursing home in Brooklyn presented this example in a class presentation where she conceptualized the role of group services within a residential facility as a means to help people who are making significant life transitions:

Well, you can say that when people come to our nursing home, it is really their last stop. Most of the people are old, although we have a few people as young as 28, but they aren't going to be going anywhere either. I had been doing what Dr. Goodman told us was "creative hanging out"–you know, just watching and listening to people to figure out what kind of group might be good. I could see pretty quickly that people who were coming in were pretty isolated, so I talked to my supervisor about beginning a newcomers' group to help people learn about the facility and make new friends. She said, "Great," but when I was trying to plan for the group she kept asking me what I was doing and why I wasn't getting started. So one day she just up and announced a group at Community Meeting. She told me a sure way to get people to come was to have food, so she announced there was going to be food and anyone could come. The first session was a flop, because the people who did come where people who were friends and had already been there a long time. They only came for the food.

I went back to the supervisor to tell her what happened and brought all my stuff from group work class about planning. I did remind her that the people who were having trouble were new and seemed isolated. I told her I thought the facility needed to help people get more integrated into our programs and that I thought the group could help. Finally, she "got it" about the purpose and understood that I would have to go around and meet with people to find out what they needed and do the other planning steps. The group worked out wonderfully.

This group worker saw the group she was proposing as consistent with a social-functioning type organization, even though the residents were living in a restrictive setting that afforded them little control over their daily lives. The socialization function of the group was meant to address a life transition from living in the community to residential care. She captured the need that the clients had in these circumstances to adjust to a new way of life. She was able to connect the client need to agency need for the supervisor and promote "collaborative learning" with her superior.

A significant change in the human service environment that remains outside of Glasser and Garvin's model is the proliferation of for-profit agencies. Every new advanced group work practice class has had at least one student employed in a setting where the overarching purpose of the agency is to make a profit. When students talk about these agencies, they call them "companies," and are aware that the services their employers offer are shaped by a profit motive. These organizations tend to merge function as both social conflict and social functioning operations. They accept referrals from community courts, alternative to incarceration programs, or services that are court mandated. In addition, they market programs to people who are voluntarily seeking treatment (often substance-abuse treatment) and offer an array of group and individual services presumably to meet to demands for these services by social control organizations.

In one class example the student-worker described her leadership team as an "autocracy" that used absolute and dictatorial power (Morgan, 1998). She described the managers as "paternalistic." The role of the group worker, who represents an authority with power to reward or sanction behavior and participation parallels the relationship between management and employees.

The agency in the class example accepts both mandated and self-referred clients and also serves clients referred and monitored by employee-assistance programs. Clients in this organization are not assigned to group services based on voluntary, involuntary, or mandated status. Instead, they attend groups based on a tiered system of recovery that uses length of sobriety or abstinence as the determining factor. As a result, group composition is heterogeneous, creating a polyglot of social control, social transition and re-socialization membership. In her analysis the student-worker found that the voluntary clients display a superior attitude over the involuntary and mandated clients, identifying them as "street people" with less motivation and insight. Although the clients all share substance abuse as a problem and are at approximately the same level of recovery, differences in their referral status overwhelms the possibility of identifying a shared need.

The proliferation of organizations that are providing social services through corporate for-profit entities is an important area of concern for social group workers. It is not clear yet how workers in these settings will be able to practice social group work. Promoting cognitive behavioral approaches with highly trained workers may provide one route to high-level professional work, but particularly since unique training in cognitive behavioral group work practice is also deficient (Rose, 2004), it may not meet standards. People interested in group work excellence may be challenged by this organizational type. The determination of class members working in these settings to leave upon graduation does not bode well for the infusion of substantial group work services.

CONCLUSION:
SKILLS FOR ORGANIZATIONAL INTERVENTION

The first requirement for group workers is to help their clients receive appropriate services. Where they encounter organizational obstacles, their professional objective should be to change social structures that limit appropriate group work services. Insight into organizational function can help group workers identify feasible ways to negotiate such problem situations (Wood and Middleman, 1989). Although class members discuss risks to professional advancement (either as interns or employees) as a limitation, this course attempts to promote skills that enable them to understand how the practices they want to promote must be consistent with the function of their service venue.

In cases where student workers have been successful in promoting group practice, they have followed the advice of Wood and Middleman (1989) and proceeded from the assumption of least contest. Progress occurs when they identify and apply strategic behavior. Gaining organization insights can help them translate the pressures they experience into new sets of ideas about practice, exploring alternative courses of action and their alternatives (Wood and Middleman, 1989).

Group work education today is incomplete if it does not prepare students for the realities of the field. Once they move past the relative protection of the field practicum, graduates should know what to expect and how to respond to the discrepancy between their experiences in school and fieldwork and the current realities of group work agency practice. The complete education of group workers should include content about the organizational context in which they will practice and techniques and skills to manage contemporary issues.

Four years of experience with student employees in this course confirms negative reports about the state of contemporary social group work. Diminishing resources for social welfare programs and the current flood of generalist practitioners may require adjustments in the education of group practitioners. When probed about how they meet real life practice dilemmas, students demonstrate persistence and optimism about social group work and seek to discover ways to use group work skills at a micro level to promote good group practice in their work settings. Introducing an organizational framework also encourages workers to move from a parochial approach in addressing problems and can help students to contemplate agency function as an opportunity as well as constraint in their work.

REFERENCES

Bergart, A. and Simon, S. (2005). Practicing what we preach: Creating groups for ourselves. *Social Work with Groups*, 27(4), 17-30.

Birnbaum, M. and Auerbach, C.(1994). Group work in graduate social work education: The price of neglect. *Journal of Social Work Education*, 30, 325-336.

Birnbaum, M. and Wayne, J. (2000). Group work in foundation generalist education: The necessity for curriculum change. *Journal of Social Work Education*, 36, 347-356.

Bitel, M. (2005). Groups in contemporary practice settings: A review of the literature. Unpublished doctoral paper. Hunter College School of Social Work, New York.

Brandler, S. and Roman, C. (1999). *Group work: Skills and strategies for effective interventions*. Binghamton, New York: The Haworth Press, Inc.

Doel, M. and Sawdon, C. (1995). A strategy for groupwork education and training in a social agency. *Groupwork*, 8(2), 189-204.

Doel, M. and Sawdon, C. (1999). No group is an island: Groupwork in a social work agency. *Groupwork*. 11(3), 50-68.

Garland, J. (1992). Developing and sustaining group work services: A systemic and systematic view. *Social Work with Groups*, 15(4), 89-97.

Garvin, C. (1984). The changing contexts of social group work practice: Challenge and opportunity. *Social Work with Groups*, 7(1), 3-19.

Gitterman, A. (2004). The mutual aid model. In Garvin, C., Gutierrez, L., and Galinsky, M., eds. *Handbook of social work with groups*. New York, New York: The Guilford Press, 93-110.

Glasser, P. and Garvin, C. (1976). An organizational model. In Roberts, R. and Northen, H., eds. *Theories of social work with groups*. New York: Columbia University Press, 75-115.

Goodman, H. (2002). Multi-family groups in the treatment of severe psychiatric disorders. *Social Work with Groups*, 24(4), 90-93.

Goodman, H. and Munoz, M. (2004). Developing social group work skills for contemporary agency practice. *Social Work with Groups, 27(1), 17-33.*

Hines, L. (2005). Evolution of group work education in social work. *Dissertation Abstracts International* 65(08A).

Kurland, R. and Malekoff, A. (1998). From the editors. *Social Work with Groups*, 21(1/2), 1-3.

Kurland, R. and Salmon, R. (1998). Caught in the doorway between education and practice: Group work's battle for survival. Plenary Address, 24th Annual Symposium of the Association for the Advancement of Social Work with Groups, Brooklyn, NY.

Kurland, R. and Salmon, R. (2002). Purpose: A misunderstood and misused keystone of group work practice. *Social Work with Groups*, 21(3), 5-16.

Kurland, R. and Salmon, R. (2003). The survival of social group work: A call to action. Plenary Address, 25th Annual Symposium of the Association for the Advancement of Social Work with Groups, Boston, MA.

Middleman, R. (1990). *Group work and the Heimlich Maneuver*. Plenary Address, 12th Annual Symposium of the Association for the Advancement of Social Work with Groups, Miami, Florida.

Middleman, R. and Wood, G. (1990). *Skills for direct practice in social work*. New York: Columbia University Press.

Morgan, G. (1998). *Images of organization: The executive edition*. San Francisco: Berrett-Koehler Publishers.

Newmann, E. (1999). Pearls in the muck. *Social Work with Groups*, 23(3), 19-36.

Nezlek, J. and Brehm, J. (1975). Hostility as a function of the opportunity to counteraggress. *Journal of Personality*, 43, 421-433.

Northen, H. and Kurland, R. (2001) S*ocial work with groups*. New York: Columbia University Press.

Rooney, R. (2004). Involuntary groups. In Garvin, C., Gutierrez, L., and Galinsky, M., eds. *Handbook of social work with groups.* New York, New York: The Guilford Press, 212-226.

Rooney, R. (1994). *Strategies for work with involuntary clients.* New York: Columbia University Press.

Rose, S. (2004). Cognitive-behavioral group work. In Garvin, C., Gutierrez, L., and Galinsky, M., eds. *Handbook of social work with groups.* New York, New York: The Guilford Press, 93-110.

Steinberg, D. (1999). Some findings from a study on the impact of group work education on social work practitioners' work with groups. *Social Work with Groups,* 16(3), 23-39.

Strozier, A. (1997). Group work in social work education: What is being taught? *Social Work with Groups,* 20(1), 65-77.

Tanenbaum, S. (2005). Evidence-based practice in mental health: Three controversies and a caveat. *Health Affairs,* 29(1), 163-173.

Tropp, E. (1978). What ever happened to group work? *Social Work with Groups,* 1(1), 85-94.

Wood, G. and Middleman, R. (1989). *The structural approach to direct practice in social work.* New York: Columbia University Press.

Purpose:
A Misunderstood and Misused
Keystone of Group Work Practice

Roselle Kurland
Robert Salmon

SUMMARY. This paper examines the use of Purpose in social group work practice. It identifies and discusses six common mistakes that practitioners often make in regard to this central concept. A group example is used to illustrate the paper's content. The paper's intent is to enhance workers' understanding of and ability to use Purpose skillfully in their work with groups. *[Article copies available for a fee from The Haworth Document Delivery Service: 1-800-HAWORTH. E-mail address: <docdelivery@haworthpress.com> Website: <http://www.HaworthPress.com> © 2006 by The Haworth Press, Inc. All rights reserved.]*

KEYWORDS. Group work, planning, client need, group purpose, group goals, group content

Originally published in 1999, *Journal of Teaching in Social Work*, 19(1/2), 123-137. Reprinted with an introduction by Robert Salmon.

This paper was originally presented at the 19th Annual Symposium of the Association for the Advancement of Social Work with Groups, October, 1997, Quebec City, Canada.

[Haworth co-indexing entry note]: "Purpose: A Misunderstood and Misused Keystone of Group Work Practice." Kurland, Roselle, and Robert Salmon. Co-published simultaneously in *Social Work with Groups* (The Haworth Press, Inc.) Vol. 29, No. 2/3, 2006, pp. 105-120; and: *Making Joyful Noise: The Art, Science, and Soul of Group Work* (ed: Andrew Malekoff, Robert Salmon, and Dominique Moyse Steinberg) The Haworth Press, Inc., 2006, pp. 105-120. Single or multiple copies of this article are available for a fee from The Haworth Document Delivery Service [1-800-HAWORTH, 9:00 a.m. - 5:00 p.m. (EST). E-mail address: docdelivery@haworthpress.com].

INTRODUCTION

When group work students and workers become involved in pre-group planning and group formation, certain principles and concepts are seen as being so important that they have achieved the stature of a mantra. Clarity of purpose is such a concept. However, as stated in the first sentence of the reprinted article that follows this introduction, "Purpose is a concept in group work that is much emphasized in the literature but often misunderstood or even overlooked in actual practice" (Kurland and Salmon, 1998a, p. 3).

A mantra is a mystical formula, or incantation, and perhaps that is the problem. In fact, there are specific steps that can be taken to achieve clarity or purpose. There is no mysticism. First, a need must be established for the group. Also, there has to be an understanding that the content is the *means* to be used to achieve the group's purpose. The purpose is the *ends*. To describe this in another way, content is the "what" of group work. Purpose is the "why" of it. Clarity of purpose exists when:

- the purpose of the group can be stated clearly and concisely by both clients and the worker,
- the stated purpose is the same for both clients and the worker, even if they might express it in different words,
- the purpose is specific enough to provide direction and implications for group content, and
- the purpose is specific enough so that both clients and the worker will know when it has been achieved (Kurland and Salmon, 1998b).

Roselle and I sometimes talked about which of our articles we liked the best. Our personal preferences differed and varied over time, but the Purpose article always was at the top of her list. She said it was an important roadmap, showing the way to good group work practice. She was right.

Robert Salmon

REFERENCES

Kurland, R. and Salmon, R. (1998a). Purpose: A misunderstood and misused keystone of group work practice. *Social Work with Groups*, 21 (3), pp. 5-17.
Kurland, R. and Salmon, R. (1998b). *Teaching a methods course in social work with groups*. Alexandria, VA: Council on Social Work Education.

Purpose is a concept in group work that is much emphasized in the literature but often misunderstood or even overlooked in actual practice. Attention to the development of clarity of group purpose frequently is neglected. One can get a sense of this neglect by asking practitioners: "What is the purpose of your group?" Often they will be unable to answer such a question, or their responses will be fuzzy or vague. The sad fact is that lack of clarity of purpose contributes mightily to the premature demise of many social work groups. Conversely, a clearly defined purpose is the powerful ally of group workers and members alike. It is crucial to the success of the groups with which we work.

This paper will examine the use of Purpose in social group work practice. It will focus on identifying mistakes that practitioners frequently make in regard to Purpose. A group example will be used to illustrate the paper's content. The paper's intent is to enhance workers' understanding of Purpose and their ability to use Purpose skillfully in their practice with groups. A group's Purpose is defined as the ends which the group collectively will pursue. It describes where the group will go–the group's aims and ultimate destination. Within the common group Purpose, individual group members may have specific expectations, individual hopes, and goals that they hope to achieve as a result of their participation in the group. These individual goals are encompassed within the overarching Purpose of the group. The Purpose of a group for blind elderly persons, for example, may be to help its members achieve increased satisfaction in their daily lives. Given that group Purpose, the personal or individual goal for one member may be to interact more with her family members while the individual goal for another member may be to overcome her fears of leaving her apartment by herself. "Individual goals reflect those personal needs and desires that group members bring to the group, and group purpose is the common cause that ties those needs and desires together" (Steinberg, 1997, p. 56).

Most textbooks on group work practice view clarity of Purpose as essential. (See, for example, Brandler and Roman, 1991, chapter 5; Henry, 1992, pp. 43-49; Glassman and Kates, 1990, p. 76; Garvin, 1997, pp. 2, 3, 51-55; Papell and Rothman, 1980, pp. 5-23; Malekoff, 1997, pp. 59-63; Shulman, 1994, chapter 9; Skinberg, 1997, pp. 52-62; Hartford, 1971, chapters 3-4; Northen, 1988, pp. 117-121.) Northen's statement (1988) well represents the view of Purpose that is prevalent in the group work literature. She says, "Clarity of purpose is essential: it provides the basic guide for both the workers and the members of the group. It provides a framework for the social worker's analytic and treatment activities and becomes a primary determinant of the group's motivation and focus" (p. 119). Research studies have, in fact, substantiated the importance of clarity of Purpose to a group's success. (See, for example, Schmidt, 1969; Garvin, 1968, 1969; Main, 1964.)

Given the literature's unanimity of emphasis on Purpose, the misuse of the concept in actual practice with groups is surprising. The mistakes that practitioners make reflect errors in workers' conceptualizations of Purpose and in their actual practice interventions in regard to group purpose. This paper focuses on six common mistakes of practitioners:

1. Practitioners promote a group Purpose without adequate consideration of client need.
2. Practitioners confuse group Purpose with group content.
3. Practitioners state group Purpose at such a high level of generality that it is vague and meaningless and, therefore, provides little direction for the group.
4. Practitioners are reluctant to share with the members *their* perceptions and ideas about the group's Purpose.
5. Practitioners function with a hidden Purpose in mind that they do not share with the group.
6. Practitioners do not understand Purpose as a dynamic, evolving concept that changes over the life of the group. Instead, they view Purpose as static and fixed.

THE CONNECTION BETWEEN CLIENT NEED AND GROUP PURPOSE

When the first thought about the formation of a new group comes into the mind of the practitioner, it usually is stimulated by the worker's perception of client need. It is, in fact, client need that is the foundation upon which a meaningful group is built. Kurland (1982), in her pregroup planning model, emphasizes the centrality of need as the basis for the development of clarity of Purpose. Group Purpose evolves and flows from a need that is felt and understood by members and worker alike and the mutual wish to meet this need. If need is not established, understood and accepted by members, Purpose will be based on false premises and the group will fail.

A common error of workers in attempting to form new groups is to disregard the perceptions that potential members have about what they need. Workers often formulate Purpose on their own without involving potential group members in the assessment of need that is so central to the determination of a group's Purpose. At other times, workers may articulate a group Purpose without ever taking into consideration the felt needs of potential members. Even if a group's Purpose can be stated clearly, if that Purpose is not connected integrally to members' perceptions of what they want and need, if need is not identified, understood and acknowledged by members, the group is doomed to failure.

The failure may occur in the worker's inability to recruit members for the group s/he has planned. The worker may be unsuccessful in getting the group off the ground because s/he is unable to help potential members see how this group connects with their concerns, how the group might be helpful to them. Even if the group does begin, it will often disintegrate after a few meetings. Members will stop coming if they view the group as unconnected to their real needs and interests.

When a potential member is being recruited for a group, s/he may–and should–ask, "Why should I join this group? What is in it for me? What will it do for me? Will it help me?" If these questions cannot be responded to, need has not been established and no clear Purpose can evolve.

How do workers go about assessing need? Above all else, they need to "hang out" and talk with potential clients. What do clients seem to want? What are their concerns? What kinds of problems or issues do they struggle with? Workers need to also talk with persons in the community (however the community is defined) and with relevant others (e.g., teachers, nurses, parents). They need to "tune in," to "imaginatively consider," to look at what has been done before, at what services currently exist and at what is lacking. They need to look for themes, things people say again and again. Workers need to formulate some ideas and then talk with people again-potential clients, persons in the community, other workers, relevant others-to test out their tentative ideas, to see if they "click." Workers cannot begin to formulate Purpose without first knowing the need.

CONFUSING PURPOSE AND CONTENT

Practitioners frequently confuse group Purpose with group content. Often, they identify the group's content–what the group will do–as its

Purpose. They confuse means and ends, identifying the group's means as ends in and of themselves. Such confusion is evident in statements such as: "The Purpose of this group is to talk about difficulties being a single parent," or "The Purpose of this group is for members to express and explore their feelings about being caregivers of persons with Huntington's Disease," or "The Purpose of this group is to help new foster parents learn about regulations and entitlements of the foster care system."

In each of these statements, what is identified as Purpose (to talk about . . ., to explore . . ., to learn about . . .,) actually is the group's content (i.e., what the group will do). Essential to the identification of a group's Purpose is a clear statement of the ends toward which the group will strive. In what ways, for example, is it hoped that talking about difficulties will be helpful to the single parents who are members of the group? Similarly, in what ways will expression and exploration of feelings be helpful to group members who are caregivers of persons with Huntington's Disease? What are the reasons that learning about the system's rules and entitlements is important to new foster parents?

Knowing the *reasons* that they are being asked to talk, to express, to explore, to learn, and the ways in which it is thought that such talking, expression, exploration and learning might be helpful to them is crucial for the members of the groups with which we work. Members' motivation and the quality of their participation are greatly enhanced when they have such understanding. Knowing what they are going to do is not enough. They need to understand why they are doing it. Members' willingness to engage whole heartedly in the work of the group, especially at times when that work is painful or difficult for them, increases remarkably when they view what the group does and what they are being asked to do as purposeful and designed to accomplish specific ends. Having a clearly defined purpose also offers the group a tangible standard to be used in evaluating the success of its work.

PURPOSE THAT IS OVERLY GENERAL

A third mistake on the part of the practitioners is to state the group's Purpose at such a high level of generality that it means little to the group and its members. To merely say that a group's Purpose is socialization or education or therapy or support or counseling or self-help is not enough. Such statements may hint at what a group is about, but they are so global that group members cannot turn to them to find direction.

Such generality does not provide focus. It does not allow for the inclusion of the goals of individual members nor provide a structure that is clear enough to evaluate the work of the group.

The degree of specificity of Purpose may differ, depending on the theoretical approach of the practitioner. Those whose practice is rooted in behavioral theory, for example, may advocate for greater specificity of Purpose, while for those whose practice is rooted in humanistic/developmental theory a more general statement of Purpose may suffice. The authors of this paper support a middle road here, on the one hand believing that a statement of Purpose that is overly specific may unnecessarily limit a group and its members and, on the other hand, seeing a statement of Purpose that is overly general as not providing a group and its members with the direction and framework that are necessary. In our experience, however, it is the overly general statements of Purpose that predominate.

Within such general purposes as socialization or therapy or support, it is necessary to define the meaning of these terms for the particular group with which one is working. The practitioner needs to ask her/himself what socialization or therapy or support would really look like in the particular group and for the particular group members with whom s/he is working. Socialization in one group, for example, might mean helping members to be able to more effectively listen to and interact with their peers, while in another group it might mean helping members to express anger and assert themselves in more constructive ways. Defining the meaning of a broad term such as socialization for a particular group and its members has important implications for the group's content. It also allows both the practitioner and the group members to know when the group's Purpose is being achieved. Thus, a statement of Purpose that has real meaning for a group and its members can serve to spur members toward its achievement.

RELUCTANCE OF THE WORKER TO SHARE IDEAS

A fourth mistake that practitioners often make in regard to Purpose is not to share their thinking about the group's Purpose with the group members. Instead, workers often ask open-ended questions of the group, such as, "What do you think the Purpose of this group should be?" Often, they then sit quietly and say nothing while members struggle among themselves to figure out the group's Purpose. Such lack of help from the worker usually results in long and highly uncomfortable silences among the group members, especially in the beginning stage of the group, or alternatively may evolve into lengthy exploration, bargaining and confusion as goals are discussed. Direction and guidelines are essential when group members need the help of the worker, especially in the beginning stage of the group.

Some workers refrain from sharing their ideas about Purpose because they do not wish to impose upon the group and believe that for a group to truly belong to its members the defining of Purpose needs to be done solely by the members. Other workers believe that the members benefit and learn from their struggle, unassisted by the worker, to define the group's Purpose. We disagree with such viewpoints. Such practice, as we see it, represents a misunderstanding and misuse of the concept of client self-determination (Kurland and Salmon, 1990) as well as a misuse of worker authority.

We envision the worker's role as an active and participatory one, especially in the group's beginnings. If the worker has done the thinking necessary to plan and form a group, then it is probable that s/he has a vision for the group and ideas about the group's Purpose. To share those ideas with the group and the thinking that gave rise to the group's formation is a way of including the members and, in fact, can help the group members to share their own thinking and ideas. Rather than imposing upon the group members, such sharing of her/his vision for the group on the part of the worker can serve to stimulate the thinking and the ideas of the group members. Perhaps the *art* of social work practice for the worker involves the use of self (through one's choice of words, tone of voice, and physical stance when one expresses one's own thinking and ideas) to communicate an invitation to group members to participate fully and to let the group members know that their ideas are needed and will be welcomed and appreciated. For the worker not to share her/his ideas and thinking about the group is to deprive the group and its members of valuable expertise and input.

HIDDEN PURPOSES

A fifth error of workers is to try to draw members into a group by stating a Purpose that they think will be inviting, using such a statement of Purpose as a kind of "bribe" to get members to come to the group. As the group continues, they keep hidden the real Purpose that they have in mind, trying to sneak it in wherever possible. The worker's *real* (hidden) purpose, which goes unstated, usually is something like "the honest expression of feelings by clients about what really is of concern in their inner lives." Workers may think that once the group gets off the ground and members are "hooked," then they will be able to let the members know what the Purpose really is. Such workers may be fearful that members will not come to a group if they know the Purpose that the worker has in mind. Or perhaps workers find it difficult to state directly words or ideas that are painful and difficult.

In an effort to make the group sound inviting, workers may altogether sidestep stating the Purpose. For example, a new mother of a child born with a cleft palate was asked to join a group. The fact that the group was for mothers of children born with cleft palates and aimed to address their special needs went unmentioned in the worker's invitation to participate. Examples abound of children in school or community groups who are never told directly by their workers that such groups aim to improve their behavior in school or their interaction with peers. Instead, workers emphasize that such groups will go on trips or participate in special activities. The difficulties such children may be having are evaded and go unmentioned. And rarely do practitioners who work with the elderly share directly with members of a reminiscence group the reasons for and benefits of reminiscing in the final life stage. Workers often may not realize that being explicit about Purpose may come as a great relief to potential group participants because they are hopeful that the group will be addressing needs that they see themselves as having.

When disparity exists between the stated and the hidden Purpose of a group, the important social work value of respect for the client is violated blatantly. For a worker to state–and for the members to understand–one Purpose and then for the worker to pursue another Purpose is highly manipulative and often results in clients being labeled as "resistant" or "not ready" when they object or refuse to go along with a ruse. Blaming the client for what is, in fact, the worker's unwillingness to be direct and honest is all too common in group work practice. There is a principle involved here: *If you cannot say it to clients, you have no right to try to do it.*

PURPOSE AS A DYNAMIC AND EVOLVING CONCEPT

Many practitioners believe it is necessary to clearly establish a group's Purpose as soon as the group begins. They mistakenly think that, once identified, a group's Purpose is immutable and unchangeable. They view Purpose as a hurdle to be overcome at the start of the group.

They see it as a static concept. Such an attitude was expressed clearly by a student who recently began working with a men's group in a long-term unit at a Veterans' Administration hospital. In a group work class after the first meeting of the group, he proudly announced, "I told the group that the Purpose of this group was to help them adjust to being in the hospital. I asked them what they thought and they all agreed that that sounded good. So then we moved on." He seemed relieved to think that Purpose would cause no trouble, glad to be able to report accomplishment in regard to a concept that his group work instructor had emphasized a great deal in class.

Often, workers fail to appreciate that Purpose is a dynamic concept and that a group's determination of Purpose is an evolutionary process. Furthermore, many practitioners fail to appreciate that a group's Purpose can deepen, develop and change as the group matures. Most important, such practitioners do not see Purpose as the ally that it can be to a group's members and to its worker. When a group member asks, "What good is all this discussion?" or says, "I don't understand what the point of all this is," workers often regard such comments as threats and interruptions to the real work of the group. They fail to recognize that such questions and comments provide *opportunities* for the group members to enter into valuable discussions of Purpose that enable them to continuously clarify their needs and wants as well as their ongoing participation in the group in order to assure that their membership in the group will havoc significance.

EVOLUTION OF PURPOSE IN A DAY TREATMENT GROUP: AN EXAMPLE

The story of a group in a day treatment program for chronically mentally ill persons (Epstein, 1997) illustrates well a number of the areas that have been discussed in this paper, especially the connection between client need and group Purpose and the way in which Purpose evolves over the life of a group.

The group began as a socialization group. The worker, a second-year MSW student, was instructed by her supervisor to focus on the clients' "lack of motivation and abundant free time." This was an open group that met weekly, composed of six to twelve members identified as "seriously and persistently mentally ill." Though composition varied from week to week, the group had a core membership of eight clients whose attendance was fairly consistent. Prior to starting the group, the worker spoke with clients informally as they ate breakfast, played pool and participated in games of bingo. During her conversations with the program participants, they described themselves as lonely, bored, and lacking things to do on the weekend. As a result of her contact with the clients, four themes regarding client need were identified by the worker:

1. need for increased and validating social contact;
2. need to practice interaction in social situations;
3. need for encouragement and support in the exploration of new activities;
4. need for practical suggestions about what to do with free time and ways to initiate involvement in free-time activities.

Given her observations of need, the worker tentatively formulated the group's Purpose as she saw it prior to the first meeting of the group:

> *To motivate and encourage members to partake in constructive social activities outside of the day program, to support members as they venture forth, and to provide and generate concrete suggestions of activities and involvements that are available to them.*

The first meeting of the group, however, demonstrated to the worker that her initial formulation of Purpose failed to address the more basic and pervasive needs of the group members. In that meeting, it became apparent that the group members were unable to engage in successful interpersonal interaction. Some of the group members blurted out statements that had little connection to what was being discussed. Some laughed aloud at other members, while others said nothing. Some members continued insensitively to urge one clearly embarrassed member to talk about whether she was a going to have sex with her boyfriend. The participation of the members in this first meeting was chaotic and confused. The members did not really talk to or hear one another.

After this meeting, the worker noted:

> The purpose statement that I had formulated reflected *my* needs and goals for the clients more so than it addressed *their* developmental and social needs and goals. I came away not knowing what would make sense in regard to Purpose but with the strong sense that the statement of Purpose I had formulated was way ahead of where the clients were, for they really seemed not to know how to interact with one another and were not ready to venture far beyond

the day treatment program into other social situations, despite their saying they were bored and lonely.

The worker's experience with the group stimulated her continued thinking about the needs of the members and what the group's Purpose might be. Thus, she reformulated her conception of the group's Purpose:

> *To help members talk about their difficulties in making friends and feeling comfortable in social situations. To gain practice and experience in new social situations and to learn to cope better with loneliness and weekends.*

Though more closely related to the group members' needs, this statement confused Purpose and content and also remained overly ambitious. In the group meetings, members were unable to articulate or discuss their situations. A trip to Rockefeller Center clearly demonstrated that the members were not yet ready or able to participate in activities outside the program. Following the trip, the worker noted:

> The trip revealed that I am pushing too fast. The clients followed me like sheep and showed little interest in anything around them. They seemed scared and relieved to return "home" to the program. My aims and goals are too high or at least too early. The clients are telling me a lot about their needs, not in their words but through their behavior.

Continued experience in and with the group led the worker to a third and much more direct and succinct formulation of purpose:

> *To improve members' abilities to interact socially.*

This statement of Purpose had clear implications for what the content of the group might be. The group itself would become a place where members could learn, practice, and experience satisfying social interaction. The members' endorsement of this group Purpose was evident in the enthusiastic nature of their participation in the group as illustrated in the following process recording.

> I wrote my new idea about Purpose on the board and read it slowly and distinctly aloud. The group members were attentive and looked

as if they were trying to take in every word. Several members were nodding. Elaine proceeded to copy the statement on a blank piece of paper. . . . We spent a little while talking about the Purpose statement. Unlike the other times when I had tried to engage the group in discussion of Purpose, they now participated actively. This Purpose seemed real to them.

I explained that I'd prepared a short demonstration of the kind of thing we might do in the group, but would need a volunteer. Alice volunteered gladly. Group members were laughing because they didn't know what to expect. I described a scenario that Alice and I were going to role-play for the group. I asked group members to imagine that Alice was a client at the clinic who was very depressed. I would be playing another client who walks by her in the reception area and tries to comfort her. I emphasized to Alice and the rest of the group that Alice's character was not feeling like talking to anyone. She was simply sitting in the reception area, waiting to see her therapist. She was depressed and wanted to be left alone.

The skit unfolded as follows: I approached Alice and tried to get her to tell me what was wrong. I appeared to be very concerned, but frenzied in my attempt to elicit a response from her. When she kept her head down, I grabbed her and gave her a big hug. I then went on to tell her how I could understand how she felt and that I was having a hard time too. I began to speak louder and faster, going on and on about my boyfriend and how he hurt me and how bad I felt. I then stopped, calling, "time-out."

Group members jumped in right away with observations about my behavior and Alice's response. Most of the group members realized that my behavior was inappropriate, particularly in light of Alice's body language. Sylvia picked up on the fact that I turned the attention from Alice's problems to my own. Several group members pointed out that I never found out from Alice what was wrong, and yet I kept talking and shared a problem I was having that might have nothing to do with her. The most interesting part of the discussion centered around the hug. Alice and Gena thought that it was a nice gesture on my part. Several other group members pointed out that it was not appropriate. I picked up on this and pointed out that it is important to respect people's personal space. I pointed out that, in situations like this, when we don't know people well, we should never be afraid to ask them what they need or how they feel about receiving a hug or wanting to talk. I emphasized that asking someone what they feel comfortable with is always a good idea, no matter what the situation.

I was quite impressed with Alice's response to all of this. She said that she liked my hug and that she was the type of person who would do just the same to someone who looked upset. She reflected for a moment: "Maybe other people are not comfortable with that, though." She said something to the effect that she had never thought about that before. I pointed out to the group that Alice has a lot of warmth and affection to offer, but that she is right: that she (and others) must be careful about who this affection is offered to, and in what situations.

That the group's Purpose was now meaningful and real to the members was demonstrated by the nature of their participation in the group meetings that followed. A process excerpt from the group's eighth meeting well illustrates their involvement and interest, with one member even taking a risk to raise a highly personal concern.

I then introduced the role-play exercise that Ms. D. (co-leader) and I had prepared. I told the group that we would need a volunteer. Several people raised their hands. Ms. D. picked Elaine. Prior to enacting the role-play, Ms. D. explained the scenario to the group. The hypothetical situation we constructed was to feature Ms. D. as the "friend" who could not stop talking; Elaine, as the demure, polite, and timid friend; and I as Elaine's conscience (or, the comic-book-like "bubble" above her head, verbalizing her "true" thoughts).

Ms. D.'s character talked and talked non-stop. She asked Elaine about her weekend, but interrupted her almost immediately, telling her how she spent her weekend shopping. . . . She again interrupted Elaine and informed her that she "must" try meditation. I would interject every two minutes or so with something like: "God, why doesn't she just stop talking. I wish she would just shut up! I don't want to hear about meditation. . . . Can't she see that I'm not listening to her anymore?" The group seemed to enjoy the role-play. They laughed, looked attentive, and clapped when it was over.

When the role-play was over, a lively discussion ensued. Group members picked up on the dynamic between Elaine and Ms. D. They commented on how Ms. D. was clueless about Elaine's needs and did not listen to her. All group members nodded yes and smiled when Ms. D. asked if they ever had experiences in which their unverbalized thoughts looked something like what I had been saying throughout the role play.

The most interesting part of the group came toward the end. Lydia made a statement to the group. She said: "I feel like people roll their eyes when I talk and care nothing about what I have to say. . . . That's why I don't talk very much in this group. I often don't want to come. . . ."

CONCLUDING STATEMENT

It is a surprising phenomenon, considering the agreement on the importance of Purpose in the literature, that this concept is so often misunderstood, or neglected, in actual practice. This paper has described six common mistakes that often are made in the formulation of group Purpose. These mistakes frequently lead to the failure of groups. This paper has focused on ways to rectify these practice errors, on ways to achieve greater clarity of Purpose in work with groups, and ultimately to provide more effective service to the group members.

REFERENCES

Brandler, Sandra and Roman, Camille, P. (1991). *Group Work: Skills and Strategies for Effective Interventions.* New York: The Haworth Press, Inc.

Epstein, Elena. (1997). "The Evolution of Group Purpose." Student paper. Hunter College School of Social Work.

Garvin, Charles D. (1969). "Complementarity of Role Expectation in Groups: The Member-Worker Contract." *Social Work Practice,* pp. 127-145.

Garvin, Charles D. (1968). *Complementarity of Role Expectations in Groups: Relationship to Worker Performance and Member Problem-Solving.* PhD dissertation, University of Chicago.

Garvin, Charles D. (1997). *Contemporary Group Work. 3rd ed.* Boston: Allyn and Bacon.

Glassman, Urania and Kates, Len. (1990). *Group Work: A Humanistic Approach.* Newbury Park, CA: Sage Publications.

Hartford, Margaret E. (1971). *Groups in Social Work.* New York: Columbia University Press.

Henry, Sue. (1992). *Group Skills in Social Work: A Four-Dimensional Approach. 2nd ed.* Pacific Grove, CA: Brooks/Cole Publishing Co.

Kurland, Roselle. (1982). *Group Formation: A Guide to the Development of Successful Groups.* New York: United Neighborhood Centers of America.

Kurland, Roselle and Salmon, Robert (1990). "Self Determination: Its Use and Misuse in Group Work Practice and Social Work Education," in *Working From Strengths: The Essence of Group Work,* David Fike and Barbara Rittner, eds. Miami, FL: Center for Group Work Studies, pp. 105-121.

Main, Marjorie White. (1964). *Selected Aspects of the Beginning Phase of Social Group Work.* PhD dissertation, University of Chicago.

Malekoff, Andrew. (1997). *Group Work with Adolescents: Principles and Practice.* New York: The Guilford Press.

Northen, Helen. (1988). *Social Work with Groups. 2nd ed.* New York: Columbia University Press.

Papell, Catherine P., and Rothman, Beulah. (1980). "Relating the Mainstream Model of Social Work with Groups to Group Psychotherapy and the Structured Group Approach." *Social Work with Groups,* 3(2): 5-23.

Schmidt, Julianna T. (1969). "The Use of Purpose in Casework Practice." *Social Work,* 14(1): 77-84.

Shulman, Lawrence. (1992). *The Skills of Helping Individuals, Families, and Groups,* 3rd ed. Itasca IL: F.E. Peacock Publishers, Inc.

Steinberg, Dominique Moyse. (1997). *The Mutual Aid Approach to Working with Groups: Helping People Help Each Other.* Northvale, NJ: Jason Aronson, Inc.

"What Could Happen and What Couldn't Happen": A Poetry Club for Kids

Andrew Malekoff

SUMMARY. This essay describes the development of a classroom-based poetry club for young children attending an alternative school, a school-based mental health program, for elementary school students identified as having serious emotional disturbances. The essay emphasizes the importance of pre-group planning, contracting, and negotiating values and norms with teachers; demystifying mutual aid; integrating group purpose and academic goals; and tapping in to children's strengths to develop creative activities. *[Article copies available for a fee from The Haworth Document Delivery Service: 1-800-HAWORTH. E-mail address: <docdelivery@haworthpress.com> Website: <http://www.HaworthPress. com> © 2006 by The Haworth Press, Inc. All rights reserved.]*

KEYWORDS. Group work, poetry, children, elementary school, education, students, teachers

---

This is a modified version of an essay by the same name published in *Families in Society* (2002), Volume 83:1. Reprinted and adapted by permission of the Alliance for Children and Families.

[Haworth co-indexing entry note]: "'What Could Happen and What Couldn't Happen': A Poetry Club for Kids." Malekoff, Andrew. Co-published simultaneously in *Social Work with Groups* (The Haworth Press, Inc.) Vol. 29, No. 2/3, 2006, pp. 121-132; and: *Making Joyful Noise: The Art, Science, and Soul of Group Work* (ed: Andrew Malekoff, Robert Salmon, and Dominique Moyse Steinberg) The Haworth Press, Inc., 2006, pp. 121-132. Single or multiple copies of this article are available for a fee from The Haworth Document Delivery Service [1-800-HAWORTH, 9:00 a.m. - 5:00 p.m. (EST). E-mail address: docdelivery@ haworthpress.com].

Available online at http://www.haworthpress.com/web/SWG
doi:10.1300/J009v29n02_09

INTRODUCTION

The boys, 5-, 6-, and 7-year-olds, arrived on their separate buses for summer school. They met their classroom aides in the front lobby of Henry Chinaski Elementary School. After gathering in the auditorium, they took the routine trek down the hall to the stairwell where they climbed together. Upon reaching the top step, they turned the corner and spotted me down the hall, standing outside their classroom.

"Mr. Andy!" they squealed as they ran down the hallway, greeting me with sweet smiles and hugs that didn't quite make it all the way around me. The boys were three of the younger members of the Poetry Club, a group I started in the spring. The group lasted ten weeks, ending about six weeks ago. "Mr. Andy! We missed you, where you been?" asked Rayshawn. "Mr. Andy, look I got a new video game," announced Simon whose attention was glued to a tiny video screen depicting figures in battle.

I bent down to watch Simon direct his troops only to be interrupted by Dustin who announced, "Mr. Andy, I made a new poem. You wanna hear it?" With a wide-eyed excitement and anticipation I nodded yes, "Please, I'd love to hear your poem." Dustin began, "It goes like this . . . okay . . . I call it . . . 'What could happen and what couldn't happen.' " Reciting from memory Dustin looked at me straight in the eyes only occasionally glancing up and away, jogging the side of his brain that would enable him to recapture the lines of the poem.

What a memory! Recently in a school-wide talent show Dustin assumed the persona of "Mr. Capital," fielding questions about state capitals from an audience of 200 adults and children. Maine . . . New York . . . California . . . Nevada . . . whatever. No one was able to stump Mr. Capital. Now, in the hallway outside his classroom, he had a grateful audience of just one. "What could happen and what couldn't happen," he began

A Dog eating a bone:
That could Happen;

A Bee making Honey:
That could Happen;

A Cat eating Cat Food:
That could Happen;

A Rhinoceros eating Rhinoceros food:
That could Happen;

A Dog making a bone from a chicken:
That couldn't Happen;

A Panda eating a Monkey:
That couldn't Happen.

A Kid eating Franks with Beans:
That could Happen!

Moved by his creativity, spirit, and generosity I wrapped my arm around Dustin and gave him a squeeze. "That's terrific Dustin. Great! I'm so proud of you. That's one of the best one's I've heard."

Little boy, heavy heart, sweet poetry:
That could Happen!

A heavy heart at 6 years old. I don't think I need to detail what that means here. You know all the risk factors and stressors. I think you get the picture. How does a child deal with a heavy heart? One evaluator from the hospital noted that Dustin has imaginary friends and is preoccupied with death.

THE INTENSIVE SUPPORT PROGRAM:
A SCHOOL-BASED MENTAL HEALTH PARTNERSHIP

The Intensive Support Program (ISP) is a partnership between a school district and a mental health center. Prior to being referred to ISP the students were either in psychiatric hospitals or considered at-risk for placement in costly long-term out-of-home institutional settings. A goal of ISP is to prevent long-term placement and help students to stay home and get an education. The program aims to normalize their growing up years, not only geographically but programmatically through strength-based interventions. Group work is a key component of ISP. Purposeful group participation offers students an opportunity to belong and feel competent and provides an interdisciplinary staff of adults a chance to develop the bonds that teamwork requires.

As administrative director of the program, I travel from our agency's central office to Henry Chinaski Elementary School and sister high and middle schools throughout the week. My responsibilities are administrative and supervisory. I try to make connections with as many young people in the program as I can. An administrative role can appear distant from frontline work. To whatever extent possible I try to prevent this, to decrease distance and mystification, by getting to know the kids through direct practice. Group work is a way to get to know several students at once and provide a needed service at the same time. In an attempt to get to know the elementary school kids and provide them with a worthwhile experience, I proposed an idea for a group, a poetry club. Then I arranged a meeting with the program social worker and classroom teachers who would be instrumental in the formation of the club. I knew that without their sanction and support it would go nowhere.

GROUP WORK IN AN ELEMENTARY SCHOOL CLASSROOM: CHALLENGES AND OPPORTUNITIES

Pre-Group Contact and Contracting with Teachers

Offering a group work service for a classroom group in a school setting presents group workers with a unique set of challenges. I knew that I needed to contract with the classroom teachers, integrate group purpose with academic and behavioral goals, and support the pro-social values promoted daily in the classroom. I thought that a poetry club could build spirit, tap students' creativity, and cultivate an appreciation for poetry that would extend beyond the life of the group itself.

The classroom composition in the program is six students, one teacher and one aide: "6-1-1 classes" is how they're referred to. At the time there were three students in each of two classes, one older and one younger. Sometimes there are additional aides assigned to individual students whose behavior demands extra support and supervision. In a pre-group planning meeting the teachers expressed ambivalence about whether the group would work. Would it disrupt the daily routine? Would it interfere with the academic goals they felt great pressure to achieve? Did the younger students have the intellectual capacity to deal with poetry? All good questions. I knew that I needed the teachers as allies and partners in order to make a Poetry Club work.

Demystifying Mutual Aid

I asked them to think about the concept of "poetry in motion." I explained that all poetry didn't have to be regimented pencil-to-paper work, and together we could help the students discover the means for finding poetic expression verbally, musically, and physically. For example, one of the group activities involved photography. Each member took turns arranging the group into their own unique tableau to be preserved photographically. I presented the idea of mutual aid as a core principle. Older students could help the younger ones and the younger ones could encourage the efforts of the older ones. The staff could easily relate to the value of promoting mutual aid. The program social worker shared a story about two of the older boys to illustrate this concept.

Davis is an overweight 9-year-old-boy who has always been teased by peers. He has a poor self-image and is convinced he will fail almost anything before he tries. He can't keep up with the kids his age who live in the neighborhood that rollerblade and ride bikes. He hasn't learned to do either.

With the help of the gym teacher, a goal for Davis was to learn these skills. Week after week Davis would procrastinate putting on the skates and helmet. Once he did he would become weepy, petrified, once standing in the middle of the gym while scores of others, younger and older, circled him. The other two members of his class teased him as the kids on his block had, telling him: "You don't know how to rollerblade."

One day as Davis stood frozen in his blades, Stan, the most athletic of the trio, zipped over to him and whispered, "C'mon Davis, you can do it." But Davis couldn't move. Stan said, "Watch me," as he gracefully glided around the perimeter of the gym. Nothing. Stan skated over and got face-to-face with Davis. He took both of Davis' hands into his and instructed him to follow his foot movements. Slowly, Davis began to move on his rollerblades. Stan let go and Davis continued to mirror his moves. Davis moved faster and faster with Stan cheering him on, "C'mon Davis. Faster. You're doing it. Keep on going."

On that day, Davis learned to rollerblade, made his first friend, and gained acceptance in the larger group as he skated round and round the gym with the other children.

Integrating Group Purpose and Academic Goals

I asked the teachers to provide me with a list of academic goals for each grade level so that they could be included in determining a mission for the group–a group purpose. It was important that the group not be perceived by the teacher as a burden, but rather as a means of assisting them in accomplishing their aims.

Below is list of academic goals the teachers handed to me (kindergarten, first, and fourth grades, representing the grade level of students in their classes at the time). This is followed by a group purpose statement that I offered and which was approved by the teachers, and later, students at a pre-group orientation meeting. It is so important to work collaboratively with teachers and respect the goals they wish to accomplish and standards they aim to maintain, if one expects to be a welcomed guest in their classroom.

Academic Goals

Kindergarten

- Grammatically correct language in complete sentences
- Participates in discussion, listens, takes turns
- Listens and follows directions
- Relates to spoken and written word
- Use picture clues for details
- Identify letter sounds
- Copy and write letters
- Print name in caps and lower case
- Express originality and inventiveness
- Comprehends a story (poetry)
- Recalls a story (poetry)
- Identify feelings and how to express them

First Grade

- Follows oral directions
- Participates in discussion
- Listens without interruption
- Listens to and enjoys story (poetry)
- Expresses feelings appropriately
- Retells story (poetry)
- Relates personal experiences
- Recognizes sight vocabulary
- Recalls important facts and ideas
- Reads orally with phrasing, expression, pacing, and volume
- Relate poetry and developmental spelling

- Use inventive and developmental spelling
- Identify feelings and how to express them

Fourth Grade

- Speaks clearly using grammatically correct language with appropriate volume
- Responds to ideas of others in conversation
- Listen for a specific purpose to gain information
- Giving the speaker one's undivided attention
- Follow the verbal sequential direction
- Express personal opinions about poetry
- Read aloud fluently and accurately
- Identify main idea and detail
- Use a variety of literature

The purpose of the group was presented as follows: The Poetry Club is a weekly group that is about learning to work together, share, have fun, and build confidence through the self expression of poetry. The goals of Poetry Club are related to academic goals including following directions, participating in discussions, and reading aloud fluently and accurately. The Poetry Club members will learn to help one another, applaud one another, and appreciate one another.

THE POETRY CLUB GETS GOING

A Ritual is Born

The Poetry Club met once a week for 10 weeks for about 40 minutes each week. After a settling-in period, the group meetings began with a reading of a "guess what poem," poetry that described something for the members to discover together: Key words were left out of the poems to create mystery. The group's assignment was to guess what the poem described. After the poem was read, the group was instructed to huddle up, like a football team might, and discuss what they thought the poem was about. Finally, when they thought they had arrived at the correct answer they would say so. The first poem was about a giraffe. An added treat was that the lines of the poem (written by Mary Ann Hoberman) were shaped as the head of a giraffe.

Giraffes
I like them.
Ask me why.
   Because they hold their heads so high.
   Because their necks stretch to the sky.
   Because they're quiet, calm, and shy.
   Because they run so fast they fly.
   Because their eyes are velvet brown.
   Because their coats are spotted tan.
   Because they eat the tops of trees.
   Because their legs have knotty knees.
   Because
   Because
   Because
   Because. That's why
I like giraffes.

And so a ritual was born: a poem read to the group, followed by a huddle with arms around shoulders, a discussion and a decision. *Fireworks*, *magic*, *clouds* . . . they liked figuring all of them out. I think they liked the huddling together and the drama, suspense, and surprise of discovering the true identity of the poem most of all. It allowed them to feel close as they attempted to reach a goal. They loved the anticipation and expectation that they deduced correctly, and the celebratory dancing and the high-five-hand-slapping that followed when they were right.

The opening ritual was followed by an assignment in which everyone was directed to create an original *guess what* poem that others would have to guess. The teachers and aides or older students helped those students who couldn't write, enabling the younger group members to create poetry verbally to be transcribed. Here's one by Rayshawn, a 6-year-old. Reader, see if you can guess what.

   It's
   Something
   That I really like
   I step on it
   I jump
   And do
   Flips on
   It.

Can you guess? A "trampoline." A "diving board?" Good try, but Rayshawn was thinking of a cartwheel. Remember this is poetry. It's not always easy to figure out. Rayshawn stumped you, but you made a good try.

After each poem the group learned to applaud and cheer. I shook each poet's hand after each recited an entry and soon the others, modeling my congratulatory behavior, did the same. Then, to add a comic twist to what would become a growing catalogue of appreciative gestures, I told them that they could give a military salute if their hands grew tired from all the applauding and shaking and slapping. And salute they did: little soldiers acknowledging their comrades in poetry.

Negotiating Values and Norms with the Classroom Teacher

At times the group members were, as I expected, rambunctious. In one instance Devin had gone beyond what his observing classroom teacher could tolerate and she pulled him aside and admonished him. Later I asked to meet with her. She explained that what she was trying to teach in the classroom, behaviorally, seemed at odds with the looseness of the Poetry Club. I assured her that I respected and agreed with the pro-social values she was teaching in the classroom. I added that I wanted to work with her to make sure that my "looseness" wouldn't compromise the classroom values. I realized that Devin's behavior itself wasn't the issue. The reprimand was really meant for me. She needed to trust that I respected her authority and would not undermine classroom standards. Only working together in this way, avoiding a defensive posture, would bring the mutual respect that would make the Poetry Club a success inside and outside of the group meetings.

At the outset of each group meeting the club members reviewed the meeting that had just past. The reviews included what we learned about how one can show their appreciation for a fellow member's effort and job well done. Applause. Hand slapping. Salutes. Soon an adult in the room suggested we add finger snapping, as in the coffee house days of the beat poets. What would be next? I silently wondered. Would they show up in berets?

The Group Gets to Work

I was pleasantly surprised the first time a teacher informed me of a poem written by a member outside of the group. It was Davis, the reluctant rollerblader. Poems-on-your-own was a practice that continued throughout the group, emphasizing that the group had taken root and was alive outside the group meeting itself. Readings of the free time poems-on-your-own, as I also referred to them, would be invited into the group. This provided positive reinforcement for the performing poets and motivation for members to practice poetry outside of the club. Davis' subject didn't surprise anyone, although no one was quite prepared for the depth of expression, talent, and ability to get to the (heavy) heart of the matter.

Friends for Now!
Once upon a time there was a snake
Who sneaked up to every frog to eat
One day he shooted from the tree
To eat the flea
He went to a frog
And said, "I'm going to eat you now"
He ate the frog
He ate it whole
So he was still alive
But he didn't realize
That he kills for no reason
So he spit out the frog
And now he has his best friend
For now!

A longer-term project was guided poetry. The members were given open-ended sentences to complete about themselves and their fellow group members probing their thoughts, interests, experiences, and strengths. The raw material was drafted as a "poem-under-construction." And each week the members would work towards the goal of refining their poem into a finished product to be included in a group ending Poetry Club journal that would record all of their work. Here's how Stan's shaped up:

Stan
Stan is excellent at sports.
I can run very fast.
He is awesome.
My favorite things to do are tennis, baseball, hockey
Football and soccer.

Stan has a good sense of humor
I like the color blue: a sad color.
Michael Jordan is a hero of Stan's
He used to be the best guy
And basketball player
He is very tall.
He can jump really high
And run fast.
He is nice.
He is a good boy.
The animal I'm most like is a cheetah: fast.
Athletic and smart and cool,
We're glad he's here and
A member of our school.

THE POETRY CLUB COMES TO AN END

The last three ending phase meetings were bittersweet with the members enjoying readings from the Poetry Club journal chronicling their good work. The younger boys in particular loved gift wrapping extra journals to bring home to their families. Free access to scissors and scotch tape was heaven for the 5-, 6-, and 7-year-olds.

The boys openly wished that the Poetry Club could continue and questioned why it had to end. Transition. Separation. Loss. Not an easy subject for the students in the Intensive Support Program.

Several weeks after the group ended, the boys made a wonderful presentation that I learned about only later. They invited the principal, assistant principals, and psychologist to hear their poems. Each was presented with a gift-wrapped Poetry Club journal.

My farewell poem to the boys, which I read to them in parting, appeared at the end of the journal.

What I'll Miss About Poetry Club
I will miss Poetry Club.
What can I do?
What can I do?

I can stand on my head and spin

Or I can think of
Dev-in;

I can stretch my arms and yawn
Or I can think of
Ray-shawn;

I can pack my bags and scram
Or I can think of
Stan;

I can make like a tornado and do the twist
Or I can think of
Dav-is.

I can flap my arms and try flyin'
Or I can think of
Sim-on.

I'll miss Poetry Club.
But now I know what to do.
I'll remember the boys
In the club by reading
This poem.

By Mister Andy

The Poetry Club living on:
That could happen.

The Meaning of Camp
and Social Group Work Principles

Lainey Collins

SUMMARY. The paper examines the experience of campers at a summer residential camp in relation to principles of group work practice that are incorporated into the camp program. Through the use of examples and stories from campers, six different principles are discussed in relation to their meaning to campers. All of the practice principles discussed are applicable to other recreational, residential, and educational settings. *[Article copies available for a fee from The Haworth Document Delivery Service: 1-800-HAWORTH. E-mail address: <docdelivery@haworthpress.com> Website: <http://www.HaworthPress.com> © 2006 by The Haworth Press, Inc. All rights reserved.]*

KEYWORDS. Activity, camp, leadership, mutual aid, social group work, practice principles, problem-solving, roles, self determination, transformation

INTRODUCTION

The first day of summer camp arrives each year like clockwork. Somewhere around the end of June, groups of campers board buses at George Washington Bus Terminal in New York City to go to camp.

[Haworth co-indexing entry note]: "The Meaning of Camp and Social Group Work Principles" Collins, Lainey. Co-published simultaneously in *Social Work with Groups* (The Haworth Press, Inc.) Vol. 29, No. 2/3, 2006, pp. 133-148; and: *Making Joyful Noise: The Art, Science, and Soul of Group Work* (ed: Andrew Malekoff, Robert Salmon, and Dominique Moyse Steinberg) The Haworth Press, Inc., 2006, pp. 133-148. Single or multiple copies of this article are available for a fee from The Haworth Document Delivery Service [1-800-HAWORTH, 9:00 a.m. - 5:00 p.m. (EST). E-mail address: docdelivery@haworthpress.com].

doi:10.1300/J009v29n02_10

Nervous counselors, fresh from days of intensive training and anticipation, greet campers as they arrive. The scene in the bus station is one of the first glimpses of what to expect at camp that session. In the chaos of departure, there is a flurry of feelings, attitudes, anxiety, and self-assuredness as campers leave the city.

Campers who have been to camp before are often calm as they wait at the station, sure that they know what to expect and who might be there. Others are loud, announcing their important status as a returning camper. "Oh, Hi Lainey! Is so-and-so at camp this summer? Do we get to go swimming today when we get to camp like last year?" New campers stand about somewhat more silently, wondering what camp is really about. Many of the parents and grandparents are full of questions, having never experienced a residential camp before.

These campers are our group members. When they come to camp, they become a member of a group, which consists of 12 campers and four counselors. Counselors are the group leaders at camp, and decisions at camp are based on living in a group and applying group work principles to situations that arise. Those principles are essential in a camp setting. Historically, group work has many of its roots in early camping programs, being places where workers found groups of "normal" individuals to work with during "leisure" hours of the day (Middleman, 1968). Those historical roots are the foundation for many of the principles of social group work practice used in the camping program today that will be discussed in this paper.

As a former camp counselor and camper, I witnessed and participated in my own growth and the growth of those individuals around me. In the camp I direct, group work principles are essential to children's experience and are incorporated into their daily life. However, I also have wondered if or how the children and staff find meaning in how principles of group work are used in that camp setting? What do they find meaningful about their experience at camp? By talking to some of the seasoned campers, I hoped to obtain their views on what was important to them at camp, and understand their relations to group work principles.

Campers returned to weekend trips during the winter months and were asked about their experience at camp. The campers stories included in this paper all come from experiences at Camp Anita Bliss Coler (ABC), one of five camps operated by The Fresh Air Fund in New York City. Camp ABC is for girls, ages 8-14, from urban neighborhoods in New York City. The only qualification for attending camp is that a family's income matches that required by schools for a free lunch. They attend camp at no cost each summer and also have the opportunity to participate in weekend camping programs throughout the year. The facility is rustic and girls live in wooden cabins without electricity. The cabins are "open-air" and are modeled after the canvas platform tents that were originally used as cabins when the camp opened in 1952. Showers and toilets are in a bathhouse that campers must walk to from their cabin. Most of the program is built around outdoor activities and nearly all of the activities occur within the group.

The campers talked most about the impact of camp in three areas that they described as being most meaningful to them. Those three areas included the sense of community at camp, the relationships they formed at camp, and the sense of accomplishment they felt at camp. In each of those broad areas, principles of group work practice in the camp environment can be identified as important to the experience of camp. The six principles that will be discussed in relation to the meanings that campers described are the importance of self-determination, the problem-solving process, mutual aid, the role of the leader, roles in the group among members, and the use of activity. Each principle will be discussed and illustrated using examples from camp and the voices of campers.

GROUP WORK IN CAMPING

Group work, prior to the development of a professional field of social group work, is a movement that began with the agencies and individuals that believed in offering services to people in group settings, such as settlement houses (Phillips, 1957). Group work in camping occurred alongside this movement and thrived in camps beginning in the 1930s because camps came ready-made with small groups (Collins, 2003). Camps offered not only small groups, but were also away from home, included the benefits of the natural environment, and provided an opportunity to create a new community (Schwartz, 1960a). Those elements that exist naturally at camp were seen as intrinsic in group work.

In 1937, Louis Blumenthal described group work in camping as the "conscious, directive force, generated by the inter-actions of leader, camper, and group, which aims at the creation of a dynamic environment that will provide opportunities for the constructive release of the powers of the individual and the group" (p. 3). He called for the utilization of the small group and the emphasis of group work in camps. As a result, Blumenthal (1948) later identified three areas in camping that he considered significantly changed as a result of the emphasis of group work in camping. According to Blumenthal, camps surveyed were more thoughtful about the use of groups in camps because efforts were made to decrease the size of camp groups, give more counselor attention to campers, and the idea of "group camping" had replaced "mass camping" in many of the camps (p.12). These were significant changes.

Group work was also emphasized in camps through the ideals set forth in the progressive education movement. Pioneers in the field of education in the late 1920s and early 1930s saw the summer camp as an opportunity for the use of "purposeful, related experiences" as a way of encouraging campers to participate in a community at summer camp (Sharp, 1930, p. 36). This included the use of the group at camp as the primary aspect of a camper's experience. Camping advocates during this time recognized that the physical distance from home environments created and the opportunity for the same group of children to interact together over time created great opportunities for group work (Smith, 2002).

In more recent camping literature, the use of groups has also been highlighted as instrumental in camps. Brower and Brower (1980) focus three out of five of their propositions about good camps on the use of groups. Those propositions include "(1) the group experience is the essence of camping, (2) groups influence behavior and enhance mental health, and (3) knowledge of group dynamics can influence camp outcomes" (p. 21). Groups at camp have been described as the most important aspect of camp because it is in the group where the real exchange about what matters occurs and where real social learning takes place (Goodrich, 1979; Halliday, 1991). A philosophy of camping called "decentralized camping" was developed based on the idea that camps should be group focused, should be based in nature, and campers should have a say in developing their own program (Goodrich, 1959).

Early on in camping, the importance of group work was recognized. It has been suggested that camping programs are still settings that are effective for social group work (Collins, 2003; Mishna et al., 2001). The principles of practice presented in this paper illustrate a current example of social group work in a specific camp.

PRINCIPLES OF GROUP WORK PRACTICE

Self Determination

In a 1998 research study on camps, it was found that camps that involved campers in decision making and planning their own camp experience had a more positive effect on campers (Marsh, 1998). Similarly, the use of self-determination in group work is important. Self-determination is used by group leaders to provide structure and guidance for individuals in a group while also encouraging members to express their own feelings and ideas (Kurland and Salmon, 1992). The idea that a group member should have a say in what happens to them in a group is important in encouraging their participation and the idea that they "own" the group.

At camp, the purpose of living in a small group is discussed on the first day. Groups that are recreational in nature, like camp, but have no discussion of purpose and content ignore the importance of self-determination on the part of group members (Northen and Kurland, 2001). Including campers in the reasons why they are at camp, in planning the daily group schedule, and in making choices about what activities they will participate in and what kind of food they will cook on their group camping trip are inherent in the camp program. Campers begin their first day of camp planning activities with their group and creating a program that they will follow. Freedom and independence are expressed as important at camp because campers have the ability to make choices and have some say in their own experience. A camper who does not want to participate in an activity often can choose an alternative activity or take on a different role in an activity. For example, a camper who does not want to participate in sports may learn to referee or keep score, which are both jobs that serve important functions. Samantha described the idea that "we have choice here" as important to the way that she feels as a camper at camp, especially one who does not enjoy running and playing sports.

Problem Solving

The camp environment has values that are different from those experienced in a large urban environment and become quickly accepted as part of the way things are done at camp. Older campers see the difference between "up here" and what is acceptable as opposed to what they are used to at home. In a discussion with older campers about fighting in their schools, for example, each camper had examples of fights in which they had participated or fights that they had witnessed in the previous few weeks at school. The conversation was lively as each camper described what had occurred or why she had chosen to get involved in the fight. When the situation was compared to camp, however, the campers immediately responded with such statements as, "It's different at camp. It's not like that." They went on to say that would never do the same thing at camp because they felt that they understood one another. "We lived together, went on a three day hike together, and know how to handle our problems with each other." Dominique describes the difference between the city and camp as, "Up here, I can trust everyone . . . and I know that certain things are not tolerated." The kind of environment at camp is important in order for campers to feel accepted and to accept themselves. That environment is also important to incorporating a meaningful problem-solving process when problems do occur.

The problem-solving process used at camp is taken directly from the process as it is described by Northen and Kurland (2001) and includes the following steps: (1) the recognition or even sensation that a problem exists, (2) problem identification, (3) problem exploration, (4) identification of possible solutions, (5) selection of a solution, (6) trying out the solution, and (7) evaluating the results (p. 192). At camp, this process is used with campers, staff, and groups and used to discuss problems in a group, between or among individuals, and among staff teams as well.

Campers talked about a change in their behavior as a result of how problems are dealt with at camp. They described the process as different to what they are used to at home where they may fight or just not talk to someone with whom they are angry. For instance, Kim, an older camper, described the process as one that is difficult at first because "no one ever made me sit down and talk about my problems with a group before." One camper described a change in herself and said that the way she handles problems at home had been noticed by her mother:

> One thing about me is that I bloomed into a social butterfly now, because I used to be real mean. My mother says it was like I was born again because I was real mean to other kids and I used to want to fight all of the time and now I don't want to do that. I don't start problems anymore because I just have a different view because of camp.

Another camper pointed out a change in her as a result of meeting different people at camp, dealing with problems in different ways, and thinking about her own behavior and how other people viewed her:

When I was younger–I don't know–for some strange reason I was a hothead. I mean I'm still the same but it's not the same. I feel I'm more mature and I carry myself totally different. You know, it was straight attitude for no reason when I was younger. Now I'm not doing that; all that was not necessary at all. What I'm saying basically is (that) camp has changed me because I've realized I was bad and people didn't like me. I'm really a nice person and people didn't see that and, you know, I really need to just grow up.

This change in behavior from what the camper perceives as "bad" to behavior that is "nice" is equated to the camper's experience at camp.

Mutual Aid

Gisela Konopka (1963) refers to three important principles of group work practice that are linked to the development of mutual aid. Those three principles are essential at camp. They are the acceptance of everyone in the group along with their strengths and weaknesses, the support of individuals in the group to form relationships that are helpful, and the support of each member to participate in the group and grow in that process. The mutual aid process has also been described as "an alliance of individuals who need each other, in varying degrees, to work on certain common problems" (Shulman and Gitterman, 1994, p. 14).

The type of community that exists at camp supports mutual aid at camp. Sara, an older camper who has only been at camp for two summers, describes the camp environment as, "We are way open here. It's like there's no rumors. No one is going to go home and say, 'Oh, she did that and she did this.' " A more open environment allows for easier relationship building because campers don't worry about who is talking about them behind their backs. The group also maintains a certain level of confidentiality, described by one camper as, "What we say here stays here." Relationships with peers at camp are important to campers. Many campers described friendships that they made at camp as some of their most important and often the reason why they return for many summers. Friends at camp are described as different than friends in the city, they are "more real" and "know them better." One camper describes this closeness that they feel to camp friends through the way that she communicates. Diamond, who has been friends with Tina at camp since they were young, explains the difference between her relationship with Tina and other friends at home. With Tina, Diamond feels like she can "say something quickly to Tina that will take me a week or two to explain to my friends at home." Part of talking to friends at home is needing to "rephrase" everything so that they can understand.

The ease of communication at camp and the prospect of being quickly understood are associated with the amount of time that they spend with each other while at camp. Part of the reason for this bond is that they are with each other in a small group "24 hours a day." What this results in often is that "you know more about the person you lived with at camp than your friend at home." The act of sharing a cabin together and eating together are attributed to these closer bonds. Friends at home are different because at camp, "when you live with a person, you find out more about them like what they're scared of, what they like, and what they don't like." One camper who has been at camp for five years explains that her friends at camp are important because, "At home I don't have anybody to talk to. When I go to camp, a lot of people like me." Other campers describe their friendships at camp as being closer than the ones at home because, "I tell people at camp a lot more than I tell my friends at home."

The relationships that campers develop among themselves as a result of living together as a group create bonds. Camp also encourages and provides opportunity for mutual aid through the shared experience of activities. Campers on a three-day hike describe moments where they couldn't have "survived" without other campers. "Remember when I fell down the hill? I couldn't have gotten up without Layla's help." Others describe experiences when they are homesick and how a fellow camper talked to them and made them feel better.

Role of the Leader

The importance of the role of the staff member at camp has been discussed in early camping literature (Brower and Brower, 1979; Goodrich, 1959; Middleman and Seever, 1963; Sharp, 1930). One description of the importance of staff says, "In the intimate relations of camp, where adults of understanding and skill may bring a detached, objective point of view to a youngster's problem, the boy or girl who is groping for something he doesn't comprehend is often started on the road to self realization" (Webb and Webb, 1953). This relationship is essential to a camper's experience. Staff at camp are also essential to the application of social group work principles in camp. William Schwartz (1960b) describes the stages at camp as being a frenzy of activity that fast-forwards quickly to middles. For that reason, beginnings are essen-

tial to camp in creating a sense of community. When a camper first arrives at camp, she is assigned to live with a group of other campers. She
meets her counselors, moves in to her cabin, and begins to learn about
the other campers that she will be living with and what the group will be
doing. Camp staff are responsible for this introduction to camp, for the
development of norms, and for helping campers begin to make connections with each other. Campers begin to have some understanding and
say in how they will be treated and will treat others at camp. The expectation is that everyone in the group participates and is free to express
themselves. How the campers perceive the initial meeting is essential to
their experience at camp.

The informal nature of the camper-staff relationship is beneficial in
creating a bond. Campers feel more open to talk to and express themselves to staff. Staff that had a positive influence on campers were described as more informal, funny and full of energy, and more attentive.
The relationships with staff at camp that are positive involve staff who
interact with campers and are energetic. Campers that were more apt to
participate in activities did so because they had a counselor that participated. "She won't have to tell you to participate; she'll just do it and
you'll see her doing it and you'll think it's fun." When campers describe
staff who were meaningful to them, they would often laugh as they recalled stories from the summer. Brittany, Denise, and Christine all rem-
inisced about some counselors they had shared the summer before.

"She was hilarious," said Brittany, laughing.
"She was funny, she was crazy. She used to make people laugh,"
Denise added.
"Remember we used to laugh because Ellen would sing about her
love for glazed doughnuts?" asked Brittany.
"She was funny," said Christine.
"And Elizabeth had that one dance that she did through the whole
thing," Brittany said.
"Yeah, the whole encampment," said Arielle, smiling.

The importance of play and humor is central to how campers respond
to their counselors and how they remember them.

Campers described staff who were more informal as easier to get to
know and more understanding. The more informal use of first names at
camp and the fact that, when addressing staff at camp, "You don't have
to call them Ms. or Mr." is important to campers in creating an easier,
less formal relationship. "Adults at camp act like us. I mean adults out-

side of camp say, 'Go sit down,' and, 'Do this and do that.'" For camp-ers, there is a distinction between school where, "You can't talk when the teacher's talking and you have to raise your hand for things," and camp, where there is a constant and free interchange between the adults and the children.

Camp is also a place where campers found counselors who talked to them, listened to them, and noticed when something was wrong. A camper, reflecting on her first summer at camp, remembered how her counselor talked to her. "She didn't talk to me like I was small, but just made me feel comfortable around here." The staff were able to let campers know when they were doing well and when they were not. Angel, who had many ad-justment problems at camp, found it helpful when her counselor was "hon-est" with her and pointed out problematic behavior to her. Staff at camp are clearly important to the experience of campers.

Roles at Camp

Camp has been described as a "transformative" experience for children who attend them. Stories from early camps describe the changing roles that campers experience as the taking of a nickname at camp (Paris, 2001). Those nicknames were attributed to the "power of camps to permit new roles and identities" (p. 60). Similarly, campers at Camp ABC described the new roles that they found at camp as meaningful to them. In the devel-opment of a group, members will take on roles that contribute in both posi-tive and negative ways toward the growth of the group (Northen and Kurland, 2001). At camp, the group provides the container in which camp-ers can try out different roles than they may play at home and at school.

Acceptance is one of the most important aspects of camp described by campers. It includes not only feeling a sense of belonging to a group but also feeling able to be different from other people and to be oneself. Campers describe the differences between themselves and the roles they play in the city and at camp as being related to how well they think they "fit" in those environments. Lisa describes the difference between how she relates to friends at school and to friends at camp as based on how she feels she can fit in.

> When I was in school, we all had a uniform and we all wore the same thing, but mentally and personality wise I always thought I was different. I came to camp and they are all different, so I felt like I could be different. People in school still call me "Oreo" because I only wear gold earrings and I listen to rock

and roll and things like that. I always felt bad and I had to hold stuff back at school, but not at camp. My friends, we'd talk in recess and they'd name their favorite artists and I couldn't say Bon Jovi or they'd look at me like, "What?" I would have to go along with my friends and say something like Ja Rule to be accepted.

The idea that Lisa had to make up things at school about herself in order to fit in is in contrast to the acceptance that she describes in the camp because she is able to be different. The school uniform epitomizes for Lisa the experience that at school everyone was the same and that there is a certain way that you should act. At camp, her role matches the role that she would like to have in the city but doesn't feel that she can because of pressure from peers.

Clothing and what campers are expected to wear in the city are also related to different roles campers play at camp. The emphasis on clothes in the city doesn't matter in camp because, "At camp you can mismatch your clothes and no one cares." There is a clear distinction made between what is acceptable at camp and what is acceptable in the city. In describing camp clothes, it is clear that, "If you go home like that, people say, 'You're crazy.' " What you are allowed to wear at camp as opposed to the city is also true for what you can say at camp and how you can act at camp as opposed to the city. For Danielle, the difference between her all-girls Catholic school that is "prim and proper" and camp are clear–at school, "if you say the wrong thing, you're dead." There are clear distinctions in knowing that "At school I cannot act the way I act at camp." Campers feel freer to share who they are with other people at camp without feeling judged.

Campers are also able to notice differences in each other after spending time together at camp. Those differences can point to a different role that a camper may play in the city as opposed to at camp. A group of campers who have been in the same camp group for several summers make the following observation about one camper during a discussion of how they saw change in themselves after camp.

Sammi: Me, a lot of things changed for me because I used to fight a lot too. Now, I control myself and I also drink a lot more water . . .

Esther: You were conceited–you remember those "bling bling" pants and you would say, "You want these?" You was mad conceited.

Ginny: Yeah, you were conceited.

Sammi: Yeah, okay, I was conceited (laughter).

The ability of campers to point out different roles they have assumed is one result of several summers of attending camp together.

This feeling of acceptance at camp is sometimes counter to the experience that campers have outside of camp. What is acceptable for girls to do at camp is often different than messages that girls get at home. For example, girls that like sports often feel more accepted at camp than in the city at school. Tiara, who for all of the years that she has been at camp, always appears dressed in clean clothes, make-up, and perfect hair, expresses the frustration with friends at home who don't believe that she wanted to work on the farm at camp as soon as she was old enough to be a Junior Staff member. She describes the reactions of her friends at home as:

> They did doubt me, mad people doubted me. They said, "What you're working on a farm? Please, you can't do it." I said, "How are you going to tell me I can't do it?" "It's just that your nails, your nails are so long," they said. "Look at you, your nails are so long, your clothes are so clean and neat, you can't do it." I said, "What makes you think I can't do it, just because I dress decent and my nails are done and my hair is so neat? What, do I have to have dirty overalls and a straw hat to be a farmer?" I guess at the end, they said she did her thing.

The experience that Tiara had after working for a summer at the farm represents the reaction campers often receive from others who respond to how they look, instead of what they can do. While none of her friends at camp questioned her ability to work at the farm, she felt questioned by friends at home because of her appearance. She felt free to try out this different role at camp even though her friends in the city doubted her ability to succeed.

Use of Activity

In working with groups of children and adolescents, Andrew Malekoff (2004) suggests that members need to feel both a sense of belonging and a sense of competence. These two things can be accomplished in a group by the use of "strengths-based" group work principles and the use of "growth-enhancing" play (p. 165). Northen and Kurland (2001) point out nine different contributions that activity can make to a group. Included in those are the ability to be creative and play, to encourage the development of relationships among members, to communicate feelings, to develop skills and increase self-esteem, and to better understand oneself and others (p. 261). At camp, the unique environment and the out-of-doors provide opportunities for children to build their sense of self-worth through participation in these activities as an individual or with a group.

The waterfront is one area of camp that was described by campers over and over again as the place where they felt a sense of accomplishment because they were able to learn how to swim or improve on their swimming. The lake, which is divided into sections with colored markers according to swimming abilities, represents for many campers a difficult area to achieve. The progression of swimming levels at the lake is one way that accomplishment is measured, as in one camper's story of achieving the highest level in swimming over a few summers at camp. "I remember the first time that I got a yellow (advanced) band. The first summer I was here, I got a red (beginning) one and then I had a blue (intermediate) band the next time. And then I tried out for yellow and I didn't think I was going to make it, but I did. When I told my mother, she was real proud."

Many campers could identify a feeling of accomplishment if they were able to move from a red band to a blue band or from a blue band to a yellow band. Many of them had set a change in swimming zones as a goal for this summer at camp. Others expressed a desire to learn how to dive or to learn how to not be afraid of the water.

Other activities at camp provide the same feeling of accomplishment. Campers describe learning how to play a song on the guitar or learning how to light a fire or being published in the camp newspaper as being among their important accomplishments at camp. One camper described her experience on the high ropes course:

> I went on the log and there were only two people to finish it–it was me and one other girl. I crawled up there and looked and walked across it like this. That was fun. I never did something like that before. I made it and I jumped off.

Campers also commented on their accomplishments at camp as:

> I felt like I was a good writer.

> You show that you have courage to actually do something in front of people.

It feels like a rush, kind of.

It's a little bit scary, but you get over it.

I feel like I've overcome something that I couldn't do before.

In the beginning it is kinda scary and after you do it you feel good about yourself and you feel like I can do this every day. You kinda boost your courage, like I can do this and I am proud of it. It kinda makes you feel good.

The impact of the camp experience intensifies with time. The longer a camper has spent at camp, the greater the effect. Campers who had been at camp for four or more summers seemed to have more insight into what had changed in them than those campers who had been there for three or fewer summers. Campers described skills that they had gained as a result of camp, including the ability to have patience and responsibility when working with others. The courage to try new things was another skill that was gained as a result of camp as well as skill in certain activities such as dance, art, and music.

Changes in how campers view themselves in the world are also noted as a result of attending camp. The voices of the children illustrate these changes:

It really changed the idea of how people are supposed to treat each other. When I went home, I didn't feel like I was being treated that way and, like, I changed my whole lifestyle and stuff like that. I moved to my father's house because I didn't feel like my mom and my family there was treating me as well as people up here. You know, like camp is up here (motions up) and everybody gotta be up there with it.

I learned confidence, I felt like I was better than people because I was a camper, I gained freedom, loyalty with friends, breath of fresh air, friendship, responsibility, acceptance, creativity, self-esteem, personal bonding, and morals, and from those experiences I gained a new outlook on daily living. That's the one thing that I try and achieve.

I saw the glass half-empty, like I saw the negative side of things, and now I see the positive side of things.

Campers see camp and their experiences at camp as changing the way that they think about and view things at home. For many, camp is a life changing experience.

CONCLUSION

Group work practice is essential in residential camping programs that seek to encourage the social and emotional growth of campers. This paper has, through the voices of campers, explored six principles of group work practice in a specific camp. Those principles of practice, emphasized in this particular camp, surface as important to the experiences and meanings described by campers.

The specific camp presented in this paper is just one example of how social group work principles can be utilized in residential camp environments. Social group workers presently underutilize camps, a setting historically influenced and heavily used by early group workers. However, it is clear that camp still presents social group workers with an arena for practice. Furthermore, as social group workers, we should continue to explore the many ways in which principles such as the ones described in this paper can be applied to the wide variety of residential, recreational, and educational systems in which we practice.

REFERENCES

Blumenthal, L. (1937). *Group work in camping*. New York, New York: Association Press.

Blumenthal, L. (1948). Group work in camping–Yesterday, today, and tomorrow. In C. E. Hendry (ed.) *A decade of group work*. New York, New York: Association Press.

Brower, R. and Brower, M. (1979). Group experience: The essence of camping. *Camping Magazine*, 52(2), 19-25.

Cohen, D. and Boblett, B. (1990). For happy campers, nothing beats the old rites of passage. *Smithsonian Magazine*, 21(5), 86-97.

Collins, L. (2003). The lost art of group work in camping. *Social Work with Groups*, 26(3), 21-41.

Goodrich, L. (1959). *Decentralized camping*. New York: Association Press.

Goodrich, L. (1979). A time for discovery. *Camping Magazine*, 52(1), 14-15.

Halliday, N. (1991). Learning through small group experiences. *Camping Magazine*, 63(8), 16-20.

Konopka, G. (1963). *Social group work: A helping process*. Englewood Cliffs, NJ: Prentice-Hall, Inc.

Kurland, R. and Salmon, R. (1992). Self-determination: its use and misuse in group work practice and graduate education. In Fike and Rittner (eds.) *Strengths: The essence of group work*. Miami, FL: Center for Group Work Studies.

Malekoff, A. (2004). *Group work with adolescents: Principles and practice.* New York, New York: The Guilford Press.

Marsh, P. (1999). *What does camp do for kids? A meta-analysis of the influence of the organized camping experience on the self constructs of youth.* Thesis, M.S. Degree in Recreation and Park Administration, Indiana University.

Middleman, R. (1969). *The non-verbal method in working with groups.* New York, New York: Association Press.

Middleman, R. and Seever, F. (1963). Short-term camping for boys with behavior problems. *Social Work*, 8(2), 88-95.

Mishna, F., Michalski, J., and Cummings, R. (2001). Camps as social work interventions: Returning to our roots. *Social Work with Groups*, 24(3/4), 153-171.

Northen, H. and Kurland, R. (2001). *Social work with groups.* New York, New York: Columbia University Press.

Paris, L. (2001). The adventures of Peanut and Bo: Summer camps and early-twentieth century girlhood. *Journal of Women's History*, 12(4), 47 - 76.

Phillips, H. (1957). *Essentials of social group work skill.* New York, New York: Association Press.

Schwartz, W. (1960a). Camping. In T. Berman-Rossi (ed.) *Social work: The collected writings of William Schwartz.* Itasca, IL: F.E. Peacock Publishers, Inc.

Schwartz, W. (1960b). Characteristics of the group experience in resident camping. In T. Berman-Rossi (ed.) *Social work: The collected writings of William Schwartz.* Itasca, IL: F.E. Peacock Publishers, Inc.

Sharp, L. (1930). *Education and the summer camp: An experiment.* New York: Teachers College, Columbia University.

Shulman, L. and Gitterman, A. (1994). The life model, mutual aid, oppression, and the mediating function. In Gitterman and Shulman (eds.) *Mutual aid groups, vulnerable populations, and the life cycle.* New York, New York: Columbia University Press.

Smith, M. (2002). *And they say we'll have some fun when it stops raining: A history of camps in America.* Unpublished doctoral dissertation, Ithaca College, Ithaca.

Webb, K. and Webb, S. (1953). *Summer magic: What children gain from camp.* New York, New York: Association Press.

Keep It in the Ring:
Using Boxing in Social Group Work
with High-Risk and Offender Youth
to Reduce Violence

Whitney Wright

SUMMARY. This article explores the concept of using boxing in social group work with juvenile offenders and high-risk youth as a means to decrease violence in their lives and their communities. It examines how learning the art of boxing can be woven into the group process to address violence. It presents ten attributes of boxing in a social group work setting that contribute to violence prevention. Examples are drawn from boxing groups in New York City and San Francisco. *[Article copies available for a fee from The Haworth Document Delivery Service: 1-800-HAWORTH. E-mail address: <docdelivery@haworthpress.com> Website: <http://www.HaworthPress. com> © 2006 by The Haworth Press, Inc. All rights reserved.]*

KEYWORDS. Boxing, violence, at-risk youth, youth offenders, identity, mutual aid, group work

INTRODUCTION

Richard sat on his stoop with the facilitator of his boxing group when a group of teenage boys walked past. "See those guys?" he said. "They're the ones I used to fight at school." "You don't fight them any-

---

[Haworth co-indexing entry note]: "Keep It in the Ring: Using Boxing in Social Group Work with High-Risk and Offender Youth to Reduce Violence." Wright, Whitney. Co-published simultaneously in *Social Work with Groups* (The Haworth Press, Inc.) Vol. 29, No. 2/3, 2006, pp. 149-174; and: *Making Joyful Noise: The Art, Science, and Soul of Group Work* (ed: Andrew Malekoff, Robert Salmon, and Dominique Moyse Steinberg) The Haworth Press, Inc., 2006, pp. 149-174. Single or multiple copies of this article are available for a fee from The Haworth Document Delivery Service [1-800-HAWORTH, 9:00 a.m. - 5:00 p.m. (EST). E-mail address: docdelivery@haworthpress.com].

Available online at http://www.haworthpress.com/web/SWG
doi:10.1300/J009v29n02_11

more?" she asked. "Nope. I don't pay 'em no mind no more. I'm a boxer."

Richard's comment demonstrates the power of self-esteem and identity in changing behavior, particularly in violence prevention for at-risk and offender youth, the underlying theory explored below. Omnipresent violence and lack of emotional support begin to tear away at the self-respect of young people. For many group members who experience violence or emotional abuse in their communities, home, schools, or from the police, the safest time in their week is at the boxing gym. Training to be a boxer taps their strengths and helps them learn more about themselves, gain confidence and find a way *out* of violence. This is no paradox: the groups take the familiar experience of fighting they already identify with and sanction it, control it, structure it, refine it, harness it, give the youth ownership of it, and turn it into an art form to be valued and respected. They recognize their new skills, talent and self-worth. By becoming boxers, they choose to keep it in the ring.

The environment inside the gym presents an alternative to their life outside. It is focused, supportive and respectful of space and others. When a young person enters the gym, he or she can embrace an engaging atmosphere and become a focused boxer. Gaining an athletic ethic through the groups helps the youth not only begin to form a positive self-identity that will help them live a fulfilling life, but it also encourages a practice of self-preservation. Engaging in boxing groups gives kids the necessary exercise for a healthy body, encourages good nutrition, and builds self-worth–a lack of which lies at the root of youth violence.

Some of the risk factors associated with young offenders that are linked to a higher probability of negative outcomes such as gang involvement, truancy or criminal behavior are lack of confidence, positive social relationships, academic ability and parental support, and concurrently living in impoverished conditions. Literature indicates that isolated or ongoing stressful events or living conditions correlate to various detrimental developmental outcomes including adolescent violent or delinquent behavior (Lerner and Galambos, 1998; Carr and Vandiver, 2001). Adolescents experiencing the above stressors are considered at-risk. Those involved in criminal behavior are considered youth offenders. Youth violent or delinquent behavior can lead to sustained criminal activity in adulthood, although many individuals exposed to such stressors and adverse conditions grow into well-adjusted and productive adults. Various factors can contribute to an adolescent's ability to transcend their environment and stop their involvement in violent or criminal behavior. Outcome studies indicate that exposure to social group work is one effective means of helping the youth develop into successful adults. Youthful offenders engaged in social group work exhibit higher self esteem, better problem-solving abilities, less recidivism and better support networks (Viney et al., 1999).

Group work has been used as an intervention modality with high-risk youth throughout the history of social group work (Northen and Kurland, 2001; Fatout, 1996; Malekoff, 1997). More recently, cognitive behavioral and curriculum-based models have emerged (Rose, 1998; Izzo and Ross, 1990; Stanton and Meyer, 1998), often eclipsing the strengths-based, mutual-aid driven work so vital for kids (Malekoff, 2001). Short-term groups have become common in recent years for many populations, including high-risk and offender youth (Mishna and Muskat, 2001). But with the fluctuating nature of adolescent behavior patterns and the attachment issues pervasive in the lives of most of these young people, short-term groups often do not provide the consistency and longevity necessary to make lasting positive behavior changes and positive identity formation.

This article presents the use of boxing in on-going social work groups of juvenile offenders and high-risk youth to reduce the violence in their lives and in their communities. The verbal and non-verbal group content helps youth to address the complexity of risk factors associated with their involvement in violent behavior. Although boxing groups can be effective for raising self-esteem, building character and reducing violent behavior for high-risk adolescent girls and boys of all ages, the following article focuses on older adolescent boys. In the model presented below, the worker is also the boxing trainer. A group worker could, however, co-lead the group with a certified boxing trainer. The model will explore youth violence, boxing for older adolescent and your offenders, group theory integrated into boxing training and ten attributes of boxing in social group work that help decrease violence.

YOUTH VIOLENCE

Homicide remains the second leading cause of death for adolescents today across the United States. Youth are twice as likely to be victims of violent crime as adults. One in three male youth from inner city neighborhoods report carrying a weapon (CDC, 2005). Three-quarters of youth convicted of a criminal offense re-offend by the age of twenty-four. Violent behavior not only poses detrimental outcomes during adolescent life, but it can significantly disrupt developmental tasks and performance in adulthood. Research has linked it to unemployment, job instability, high rates of physical health problems, drug use and difficulties in interpersonal relationships in adulthood (Borduin and Schaeffer, 1998).

The antecedents to violent behavior are complex and involve all levels of society. When the adults in their lives such as parents, teachers, action heroes or political leaders do not model positive and constructive conflict resolution, children do not learn alternatives to aggressive, reactive behavior. Aggressive children tend to assume others have similar aggressive intent and react accordingly. This internalized conflict-laden behavior develops into the adolescent perception of constant opposition to others (Franz, 2002). Many children are witnesses or direct victims of violence in their families or communities. As frequent victims, the children develop emotional symptoms that impact their coping ability. Abused or neglected children may act out to get any kind of attention at all, even negative attention. This is compounded by neighborhood violence, the regularity of which can seem to justify circumstances for yet more violence (Riner and Saywell, 2002). The result is a lifestyle that tolerates weapons, drugs, and aggressive interpersonal behavior and the invasive concept of loyalty against rivals or "us versus them." The perception of invulnerability among this age group coupled with an inadequate concept of death can prevent teens from grasping the lethal consequences of their actions (Malekoff, 1997). Therefore, a developmental cycle of negative reinforcement perpetuates an acceptance of violent behavior (Franz, 2002).

BOXING IN GROUP WORK FOR HIGH-RISK YOUTH

Service providers have long struggled to find intervention modalities effective for this population. Programs have traditionally not reached the desired rehabilitative outcomes (Borduin et al., 1995; Riner and Saywell, 2002). Older high-risk teens are often considered the most challenging population to reach, engage and retain in services (Calhoun, 2001). The youth typically spend little time with their families or at school, and are rarely open to constructive relationships with adults. Peer relations tend to reinforce anti-social behavior. Additionally, many of the teens have not had the resources necessary to build the skills necessary to fulfill their individual and social responsibilities and achieve developmental milestones.

In late adolescence, young people often pit themselves against defined rules and norms as a means of asserting control over their lives. Yet it is also the first time when youth must plan for the future. Older at-risk teens are in vital need of age-specific emotional support, self-esteem enhancement and skills to make positive decisions to keep themselves and their communities healthy and safe. For the same reason many basketball programs are successful in helping kids find pride through a positive activity, boxing provides an activity they already appreciate and admire. But self-esteem is not enhanced automatically through participation in sports, but rather through supportive interactions with adults and peers (Hodge and Danish, 2001). Though boxing programs may not have the capacity to address all the comorbid risk factors, an advantage of boxing groups for juvenile offenders is the high rate of attendance. The attendance rate provides the worker with considerable hours of face-time with members.

Many teens in the target population have not had the opportunity to complete or be a part of something they can be proud of. A lack of a sense of competence and recognition by others leads to poor self-esteem. Youth will gain a sense of mastery and pride when they engage in strength-based programming that helps them to learn a new skill and that gives them acknowledgement for their achievement (Brandler and Roman, 1991). Positive self-identity then begins to shift one's sense of self to that of someone able to take constructive control of his own life.

The concept outlined below uses an integrated approach to boxing training. In comparison to a boxing class, participants build positive relationships with each other and the group facilitator and discuss and share all aspects of learning the sport. The boxers in the group discuss the violence in their lives and how boxing has changed them. They learn tactics from each other that help them to stay safe in and out of the ring. And they gain an aesthetic appreciation for boxing as more than a sport, exercise or entertainment, but as a very challenging journey of self-exploration and self-improvement, as an art form and as the "sweet science."

Boxing groups combine boxing training with group counseling, offering a dynamic, innovative and engaging approach to services for high-risk older youth involved in violent acts. This concept is consistent with the theoretical basis and values of social work with groups: individual development through relationships with others and an underlying assumption that individualized growth and social ends are interdependent (Northen and Kurland, 2001). The sharing of ideas and experiences fosters an atmosphere for positive change.

Ample literature praises the use of activities in social group work for high-risk youth (Northen and Kurland, 2001; Wright, 1999; Gerber, 1998; Fashimpar, 1991; Fatout, 1996; Middleman and Wood, 1990). Boxing classes, as in art or poetry classes, certainly have value for acquiring skills and providing an alternative to the street for kids. Boxing groups, as any activity group, have the additional element of a discussed and agreed upon second purpose. Following the framework for the use of purpose in on-going activity groups, boxing groups maintain two separate but co-existing purposes (Northen and Kurland, 2001; Wright, 1999). The activity-oriented purpose is to learn to box. The personal growth-oriented purpose is to decrease violence in the members' lives.

The personal growth purpose is made explicit and discussed during the very first session of the group. Verbal processing takes place in the beginning of group when they put on their protective hand wraps, throughout the session during the one-minute rest time on the spar clock, and during dinner after training is over. One particularly salient guideline of group participation is that membership are not to use their boxing skills outside the group. Due to the pervasive violence in their communities and in their peer relations, members will inevitably find themselves in violent situations. They are expected to discuss these situations in full with the group to make sense of what happened, what could have happened, and possible alternative approaches to handle it in the future.

TEN ATTRIBUTES OF EFFECTIVE BOXING GROUPS

The leader's role is to teach the art of boxing and make sure that mutual aid and purposeful processing happens. The leader must weave social and personal growth into the process. She ignites the cognitive understanding of the boxing experience and helps the members to articulate how it relates to their lives and the world outside the group. Following are ten attributes of effective boxing groups that help to decrease violence in the lives of the members. Process examples for many of the attributes are provided.

1. Provides Group Members with a New Identity

The need for young people to feel valued in their community significantly influences their behavior. The developmental stage of adolescence is marked by a search for identity. Kids adopt only those identities they understand and respect. Boxing is a highly respected sport in the inner city, so a young person who becomes a boxer can adopt that identity and wear it with pride. The need to prove oneself as tough or a fighter on the street is, thus, diminished.

Since adolescence is a time of exploration, experimentation, and a search for self, any effort to make positive changes in the behavior patterns of youth needs to address the importance and strength of their identity (Calhoun, 2001). As the process of "doing" directly relates to the sense of self, activity groups provide youth with constructive paths for building self-identity (Brandler and Roman, 1991). The ultimate goals of identity formation are a firm sense of ego strength, stabilized behavior and character and acceptable roles in our communities. High-risk and offender youth are in need of experiences that socialize them into positive self-identities that highlight their strengths and support their self-confidence. A healthy self-concept will lead them to make decisions to value their life and the lives of others.

American culture underutilizes our high-risk and offender youth, especially young men. Our communities lack sufficient avenues for constructive identity formation for young males. Rarely do services truly focus on the strengths of these individuals, but rather on controlling them, punishing them or "fixing" them. Boys are also taught to be ashamed of their needs for support and nurturance, hence, introducing shame into the developing boy's self-esteem (Spielberg, 2001). As they grow into adolescents, they never develop the skills to communicate their feelings or needs, thus not receiving the support necessary for healthy ego growth.

Self-esteem is particularly troubling for African American male youth. Visible and invisible racism, neighborhood conditions in low-income communities and problems in school contribute to a sense of low self-worth. Media images of African American males as dangerous criminals or predators become internalized into young people's concept of who they are or who they will be. The group was discussing the common topic of where on their body they would want to be shot. Eighty percent of young people in their neighborhood in San Francisco know someone who has been shot (Brothers Against Guns, 2004).

Kay-O: In the leg.

J-Oh: No way, in the arm.

Kay-O: Yeah, in the arm. Jamal had it best–in the shoulder, and he's fine.

Worker: What would make you want to be shot in the arm?

Blaze: The scar but you don't die.

Worker: What about not getting shot at all?

They were silent.

Worker: Did I ruin the game?

Kay-O: Yeah, you gotta get shot.

Worker: What does it mean to you to get shot?

Kay- O: Everybody from here gets shot.

Worker: Sounds like you may secretly want to get shot.

They laughed with embarrassment then admitted people think it's sort of cool to be shot.

Worker: Okay, if you got shot and lived, can you think of how you would feel about your scar?

Blaze: Proud.

Kay-O: I could show people what my life is like, like I'm really from Hunters Point.

Blaze: Yeah, people could respect it. It's our life.

J-Oh: Like an O.G. (old gangsta).

Worker: So to be shot means to you guys that you are truly part of your neighborhood. And am I hearing that it gives you some street cred?

They all looked embarrassed again, but nodded. We discussed what street cred is and why it's important to them. Their male role models are men a few years older than they are who have been in gang disputes and made it out alive.

Worker: Is getting shot the only way to get street cred?

Kay-O: Rapping.

J-Oh: Yeah, cut a CD. Here, cut this up.

J-Oh put a CD on the boombox a friend of his had made. The lyrics depicted bullets spraying, set identity (part of the neighborhood the artists identify with) and the killings of youth from rival parts of the neighborhood. We discussed the ubiquitous violence in the music and the history of rap artists shooting each other in San Francisco.

Worker: Can any of you think of a way to be respected by your peers without the violence?

Kay-O: I get hella props for boxing.

Blaze: Boxing's hella tight.

J-Oh: Yeah, we're playas.

Worker: Playas respect each other, right?

Kay-O: And themselves.

Worker: So maybe you don't need to get shot after all to get respect from the O.G.s?

Kay-O: My older cousin tells all his friends I'm a boxer.

Worker: What's it like to be boxers?

J-Oh: Off the hook.

Worker: What's different about being a boxer than before when you weren't?

Kay-O: I'm something now. I wasn't anything before.

Blaze: Yeah, we're boxers!

They all threw a couple of punches in the air, high-fived each other then agreed that they could not be boxers if they were hurt or killed in fights. The group then discussed the moratorium on professional boxers using their skills outside the ring.

2. Promotes and Offers Safety

Boxing groups not only keep the youth off the street during after-school hours when they are most likely to commit or be victims of violent crimes (Osofsky, 2001). The groups also keep them physically and emotionally safe. "Safety is the absolute first priority in amateur boxing and training" (USA Boxing, 2005), making the group meeting often the safest time of their day.

The mutual support discussed in greater detail below adds a component of emotional safety allowing them to address issues otherwise too overwhelming. The group is a place for the members to take "safe risks" in a safe environment and to play out new and different parts of themselves (Malekoff, 1997). The reciprocity, or mutual aid, that is encouraged and strengthened by the worker provides a reality-testing base where members' ideas are accepted, confronted, and safely challenged by others. The violence prevention purpose is reinforced continually throughout the life of the group helps the group set the norm of safety in the group and value safety out of the group.

3. Provides Discipline

The notion of self-imposed accountability and consequences must emerge during older adolescence for a young person to emotionally mature into adulthood. Older youth are thus in a place in their lives when they must build skills necessary to live on their own and make important choices and judgments. Clear and consistent directions during training offers the members structure often absent in other areas of their lives. They begin to impose their own internal discipline as they grow into boxers. They can understand the need to keep training or to carry out other responsibilities in their lives and can make their own choices to do so.

Chris was taking a break during the training period.

Luis: Yo, Chris, we gotta keep going. We're sparring next week and need all the workout we can get.

Richard: Yeah, I thought about skipping group because of that game tonight, but she keeps buggin' on me about my defense. I gotta work on it before sparring. That's all I'm working on today.

4. Uses Defense as a Metaphor

The use of metaphors in social group work is well documented (Northen and Kurland, 2001; Duffy, 2001; Brandler and Roman, 1991). Middleman and Wood suggest the power of metaphors is an integral part of group work process (1985). Activity groups in particular can provide a rich context in which metaphors can harness the experience of learning an activity that connects the group to the personal growth purpose. Metaphors help to heighten the cognitive understanding in the learning process and help to relate it to members' lives outside of the group (Wright, 1999).

A pervasive metaphor in boxing groups is the defense necessary to stay safe in the ring. A boxer needs to know that he or she can be in the ring with another equally skilled boxer and be protected. When young people start boxing, they typically just want to punch–a lot and hard. But they need to learn how to make the other boxer miss. They need to see the punches coming and slip under them to not get hit. They need to stay safe in order to stay in the ring.

A mantra with offender youth is that adults are trying to "play" them–trying to get them in trouble or make life more difficult for them. This could be a teacher adding extra homework or a probation officer deciding to give a urine test. The result is often a defensive, inappropriate, and disrespectful reaction by the youth. A basic principle of violence prevention is to not allow oneself to become mad. Learning emotional defense helps the youth "slip under a punch" and not let comments–whether made by adults or other youth–engender angry responses.

J-Oh: I got kicked out of class today again. That lady, she tried to play me. She said I was messin' with this girl's hat. She does too much, I wasn't doin' nothin'. It was the girl, she was messin' with me. That's not right.

Blaze: She was playin' you.

J-Oh: Yeah, Man. She kept saying I was messin'. I didn't like that.

          Blaze and Kay-O were shaking their heads in empathic recognition.

Worker: Sounds like you might have said something to the teacher she didn't like.

J-Oh: Yeah, I told her off. She can't be playin' me like that. She always does that. She didn't say nothin' to the girl. Not right.

Worker: So you got kicked out for talking back to the teacher not for messing with the girl's hat.

J-Oh: Yeah, but she can't do that. She always does too much.

Worker: You're pretty worked up about it.

J-Oh: Yeah, I had to stay after school. I almost missed boxing.

The worker gave the other members a look encouraging them to fill in the blank. They were very familiar by this time with using boxing metaphors in their lives.

Kay-O: Oh, yeah. You didn't slip under the punch, Dude.

          J-Oh started to defend his actions by blaming the teacher.

Blaze: You almost missed boxing!

Worker: Was it worth almost missing boxing for? And still being pissed off about it?

          J-Oh shook his head.

Worker: Did you win?

          They all shook their heads.

Blaze: He got in more trouble. You should've just forgotten about it. Now she's gonna keep doing it.

Kay-O: You were all offense and no defense. You got hit 'cause you went in straight. Slip under the punch, Man, remember?

5. *Improves Impulse Control and Patience*

Adolescents, with their characteristic short attention spans, are notorious for wanting immediate solutions. Waiting to work out a conflict often does not seem an option. Long-term diplomatic solutions require work, time and energy. Controlling their impulses in the ring helps group members hold back in the moment of a conflict. Similarly, increasing their patience over the course of training helps them see long-term benefits of the time investment.

A boxer who is out of control will either get hurt or disqualified. A good boxer is precise, is strategic, and is absolutely under control at all times. Punching madly, even on the heavy bag, is not allowed. Each punch must be exact, straight, and thrown at the right time with the right combination and the right body movements. Kids want the instant gratification of letting their fists fly. If they do so, the worker stops them and makes them repeat the movement until they do it correctly. Though they begin each session eager to start punching, they may not go directly to the bag and begin training. They must first warm up then shadow box for several rounds.

When youth begin to train, they want to spar right away. Since no boxing equipment mimics the act of sparing exactly, they need to train extensively until they are ready to get in the ring with an opponent. The fundamentals, including perfect footwork, are essential to learn and can be very frustrating to master. A lot of training goes a little way. One young person who had been training for a few months said, "I want to box so bad it hurts." The youth need to sustain that desire to learn despite the dissatisfaction of waiting. If they are allowed to spar right away, they will not understand the complexities of the strategies or skill base, and ultimately not learn their fundamentals completely. Waiting to spar until they have made an investment in the sport, have begun to understand boxing and have integrated both offense and defense, helps them to value the act of sparing and to take pride in the patience it took them to get there. They are expected to apply the patience they learn through boxing to the conflicts they may encounter in their lives so verbal negotiation or other means of avoiding violence can be employed.

> The week the Iraq war began, the group discussed global violence. The members decided that the President needed to be in the boxing group.

Kay-O: Isn't he supposed to have meetings first instead of just bombing people?

Blaze: Takes too long.

Worker: Are you saying he wasn't being patient enough?

Kay-O: Yeah, couldn't he just talk it out like we're supposed to do? Or what about those NWBs? (referring to weapons of mass destruction–WMDs).

J-Oh: Nah, Bush is just trying to show how gangsta he is.

6. Develops Ability to Focus

Youth today grow up with fast action video games and movies and television shows typified by quick cuts. They are increasingly diagnosed with attention deficit hyperactivity disorder and experience difficulties focusing and staying seated in school. Whether diagnosed with ADHD or not, many at-risk youth struggle with their limited ability to focus. They describe not being able to concentrate long enough to complete assignments or follow lectures.

Boxing training is structured around the spar clock: three minutes of training, one of minute rest. During the three minutes of training, the kids may not stop. They need to remain focused for the entire three minutes. When they are sparing, if they break concentration and drop their guard, they will almost certainly get tagged.

The group was discussing the skills they have learned in boxing and if they can make direct or even indirect connection to how they have affected their lives.

Chris: When I'm in class and I'm totally bored I pretend there's a spar clock. I look at what time it is, listen the teacher for three minutes then give my brain a minute rest. Then I start listening again.

Richard: But what if she says something that's going to be on the test during your rest?

Chris: Yo, it's better than not listing at all like before.

Blaze had been working on the mitts with the worker for several rounds. He finds concentrating in school and elsewhere very difficult. During the three-minute rounds on the mitts he did not look away once or even fall out of step with the combinations the worker was calling. When they finished the set of rounds, the worker hugged him, gave him some water and wiped the sweat from his forehead.

Worker: How did you feel on the mitts for so long?

Blaze: It totally cleared my mind. Nothing else existed.

7. Teaches Commitment and Offers Meaning

With the tragic rate of adolescent homicide in our inner cities, many young people do not believe they will live into adulthood. They have lost friends to violent deaths, family members to incarceration, and various adults. For example, adults ranging from stepfathers to social workers come in and out of their lives. Their world has proven impermanent, inconsistent and unreliable. Without a model of successful adulthood, long-term goals and dreams for their future are difficult to sustain.

Adolescents who have experienced this kind of trauma and loss can have a very difficult time committing to anything or to anyone. They often do not believe the worker will actually show up next time. They also may not want to make the commitment out of fear of loss of the relationship with the worker and even loss of the ability to continue to train (loss of program or their own physical ability to remain athletic).

Once involved in boxing they can see the commitment the worker has made both to boxing and to them. They can begin to take ownership of the sport. They also see that their commitment will eventually pay off in a new positive self-identity, better academic performance, better physical conditioning, and a more enjoyable and fulfilling day. Without the commitment, the experience remains superficial, unrewarding and another disappointment in their lives.

In behavior modification theory, change takes place with the presence of skills, knowledge, community support and personal meaning. The youth may lack a reason or meaning for which to improve their lives. Many have not felt a purpose for themselves. A commitment to boxing provides a goal, something to work towards, something to stay safe for, something to have a future for.

Luis: I want to keep boxing forever.

Richard: You should get a job at the gym.

Jonathan: Maybe I can do it with you.

             Jonathan, unlike the other group members, often got picked on at school. He was not very fit or physically coordinated, making boxing particularly challenging for him.

Chris: But you don't really like boxing that much.

Jonathan: I told people at school about our boxing. The guys who jumped me have been asking me about it. They wish they could join the group.

Worker: You were the boxing expert.

Jonathan: Yeah, they think it's really cool. People aren't going to be buggin' on me anymore.

Worker: So boxing sort of means a kind of protection for Jonathan, right? Can anyone else think of what boxing means to them.

Luis: It keeps me healthy and my girlfriend likes it.

Richard: I want to be really good at it. I've never really cared that much about other things.

Chris: I can always do it. Maybe someday I can be a trainer like you (to the worker).

Worker: You're right, you can if you stick with it.

8. Teaches and Provides Respect

Disrespect–or a *dis*–may lie at the root of a fight on the street. Respect, on the contrary, is a basic tenet of boxing. Boxing requires bravery, endurance, pain, and self-exploration. The courage it takes to strap on the gloves and face an opponent–or even oneself in training–inspires respect. In amateur boxing an ethic of respect runs through the sport. At the beginning of a match, the opponents touch gloves, mimicking a handshake. At the end of a match, the opponents hug or make a similar friendly gesture, then each acknowledges the other's coach. As opposed to street fighting that arises from disrespect, boxers maintain respect for each other since they know the hard work and pain their opponent endured to get there.

> Blaze and Kay-O had just sparred for the first time. Kay-O is 30 lbs. heavier, making it much more challenging for Blaze.

Worker: How did it feel to be in there with Kay-O?

Blaze: (towards Kay-O) You're a sick (meaning good) boxer. Respect (they touched gloves).

Worker: What was it like sparring with Blaze?

Kay-O: You're fast, Man. I didn't see some of those coming. Respect.

9. Relieves Stress

Since inner city youth seldom have access to abundant sports programs and may not have grown up with a family ethic of physical fitness, they may not get enough exercise. Exercise produces endorphins that regulate stress. Acting out in school and rough housing in the halls can be a direct result of not getting enough exercise, not releasing endorphins. The youth need an outlet and often turn to fighting to relieve the pent-up stress.

After two hours in the gym, they are physically tired. They may no longer need to release that stress through conflicts with other youth. Many teachers remark on the significant reduction in acting-out behavior in school once the youth have begun boxing regularly. Parents similarly comment on the improved attitude of their kids at home, positive relationships with their siblings and reduced need to hang out on the street during late hours.

The mutual aid in the group allows the members to express intimate and often painful issues. The ability to express feelings and cope with stress serve as protective factors for young people exposed to violence (Osofsky, 2001). Exploring the effects of a violent environment on their physical and emotional well being and normalizing the physical response helps them understand the psychological reasons that often lie at the root of physical symptoms. They can also learn to manage their stress by becoming aware of how their stress manifests in their body.

Kay-O was having a difficult time loosening his body. His punches were almost perfect and his footwork better than ever. But his defense was horrible because he could not move his upper body in any fluid motion. His body was locked up. After stretches and loosening exercises, the worker asked him to talk about the stresses in his life.

> Worker: Can you think of some things that might cause stress in your life?
>
> Kay-O: Yeah, the cops keep stopping me at gunpoint. They say 'give us your gun.' Don't have a gun anymore.
>
> Blaze: That happened to me last week. I was just standing there.
>
> Worker: Can you guys think of what your body feels like when that happens?
>
> Blaze: I couldn't move. Like I was frozen.
>
> Kay-O: It's worse than having a Sunnydale dude point a gun at your face. (Note: Sunnydale is a rival neighborhood.)

The group discussed the difference between the accountability of the police for shooting someone and that of a rival. The members all agreed the police would shoot them with less fear of accountability than a rival would.

> Worker: Have any of you noticed any change in your sleeping since the police started accosting you?
>
> J-Oh: I never sleep.

Worker: What keeps you from sleeping?

J-Oh: Dunno.

Worker: Do you hear anything outside at night?

J-Oh: Yeah, but that's normal.

Worker: What do you guys hear?

Kay-O: Gun shots. But that's during the day, too. A guy got shot right outside my house a minute ago. (Note: "a minute" can mean several days or weeks.)

They discussed the guy and how they all knew him and whom they think shot him.

Worker: Do any of you think so much shooting in your neighborhood might make you feel stressed or keep you from sleeping or effect you emotionally?

They all denied that it makes them stressed, claiming it is just part of life. Then they talked about where in their body they would want to be shot (a common topic, please see process for Identity as a Boxer above). Joe added some specifics of what it's like getting shot in the belly. Their speech became quicker and more colloquial as they stayed on the topic.

Worker: You're talking about and imagining getting shot. I can hear the tension in your voices. And you do this all the time.

They kept going.

Worker: Okay. So let me get this straight. You guys all agree that people–including yourselves, J-Oh–are getting shot right in front of your houses and the cops accost you at gun point and there is no connection to your stress level?

They all became silent.

Worker: Do you think it's possible that your muscles are tight for a reason other than lack of stretching? Maybe one reason

> it's hard to relax your body in training is that there is no time during the day or night when you can truly relax? They all stared at me and quietly nodded.

Kay-O: We can relax here.

They were each finally able to admit that being "concerned" about the violence did not mean that they are not tough individuals. Eventually, they were able to drop the code word "concern" and use the word that truly depicts their constant state of being: "fear."

10. Fosters Mutual Aid

An important aspect of behavior change theory mentioned above is community support. Since many high-risk youth have difficulty forming and maintaining trusting relationships due to disappointing past experiences with adults and peers alike, attachment theory must underpin the content of the group. The likeliness of violent behavior is lessened if an adolescent forms meaningful emotional attachments with others who do not condone violence (Spielberg, 2001; Osofsky 2001). Similarly, research indicates that the strength of the alliance between youth and staff can make a significant contribution to positive behavior change (Clark, 2001). Therefore, the groups emphasize the acceptance of the youth by others, placing mutual aid at the heart of the boxing groups. As Northen and Kurland wrote, mutual aid is when "each member carries a contributing, as well as taking role" (2001). Boxers involved in the program not only get to support each other during discussion times, but they help each other train by holding the bags, watching each other's form, encouraging each other to finish a round, etc. The friendships they develop often transcend the group, increasing their engagement with pro-social peers and expanding their social support networks.

When one group needed to end, the members decided on a termination activity that they could take with them. They wrote messages to each other and the worker on each person's hand wraps. The messages included favorite memories of the group, things they learned from each other, etc. The group decided they wanted to share what was written on their wraps.

Jonathan: (Reading from his wrap) You're mad cool. You are the most dedicated one here because you don't even like boxing but you still come every time. Peace.

Jonathan started getting choked up. The group began to tease him a bit in a big brother way.

> Luis: Yo bro, keep it together. Rich is gonna come after you with that left hook.

Jonathan laughed and Chris rubbed his head. Luis began to read from his wraps.

> Luis: You are the next Zab Juda. Don't know what we'd do with out you.

Luis, the indigenous leader, also was touched by the message on his wraps.

> Luis: I don't know what I'd do with out you guys, either. I love you guys.

Sometimes mutual support is stimulated by the drama of the streets, as events unfold that are beyond the members' control. J-Oh's cousin was shot and killed a few days before a group session. Kay-O had phoned the worker to let her know about his loss. She suggested he call J-Oh to encourage him at make it to the next group. When J-Oh showed up for the boxing group he was wearing the customary laminated paper plaque around his neck with a photo of his loved one who had been shot. The members and leader hugged J-Oh.

> Kay-O: La'quan, he was a cool cat. That's gotta be rough.

> Kay-O: When my cousin died we all rented white tuxes for the funeral and wore Jordon's (tennis shoes) and those t-shirts.

> J-Oh: Good idea.

> Worker: You still wear that shirt.

> Kay-O: Yeah, it has his picture, his birthday and when he was killed. And "I'll see you when I get there."

> J-Oh: I'll see La'quan when I get there.

There was an unusually long moment of silence followed by each member talking about the young people they know who have died.

J-Oh: Any day. You never know.

Blaze: Word.

The group proceeded to discuss their feeling of fatality that they have from seeing so many people their age die. The discussion moved to their lack of self-image as future adults.

Blaze: That's why you gotta have fun now. You don't know how long you'll be here.

Worker: I want you guys to be here.

Kay-O: We know. That's why we're boxing with you.

A photographer was coming at the end of the group that day to take some photos. The members and leader huddled together for their picture.

J-Oh: Wait, should I take this off for the picture? (holding up the plaque around his neck).

Kay-O: No, man. Keep it on.

At other times, tragedies of the street reach right in to the group itself. The worker received a call from San Francisco General Hospital that J-Oh had been shot in front of his house. The bullet went through his left side, rupturing the liver. He had been unconscious for two days. After several days in the hospital he could return home with the help of the worker to change his bandages daily. Once J-Oh was strong enough, the worker brought the other boxing group members to J-Oh's house when she changed the bandages.

Worker: J-Oh, is it okay if the guys look at your wound?

J-Oh: Yeah, sure.

Kay-O: So it went all the way through? Scars on the back and the front?

Blaze: Those will be sick scars.

They talked about scars other people they know have.

Worker: Let's look at where those scars will be. Let's see . . . a couple of inches this way (she points to the middle of his back) and what would the bullet have hit?

Blaze: His backbone.

The worker nods and motions for him to make the inference.

Blaze: He'd be paralyzed.

Worker: What about a few inches this way?

J-Oh: It would've busted through my heart.

Worker: And a few inches this way.

Kay-O: You'd lose your dick, Bro.

Worker: Still think those scars would be sick?

The members talked about people they know in wheelchairs, how J-Oh wouldn't be able to box if he were paralyzed and about friends who died of gunshot wounds.

Blaze: You scared?

J-Oh: Nah.

Kay-O: I would be. Dude, you're mad lucky.

J-Oh: Yeah.

They talked about how important J-Oh is and about how many people would miss him if he had been killed.

CONCLUSION

The group context affords members the safety to admit that they do not want violence in their lives, despite the seductive nature of the culture of violence. They understand that they are not alone in their internal conflict between fear and a gangsta identity. Nor are they alone in their struggle to cope with the omnipresent violence and loss around them. A sense of belonging and universality of experience and meaning helps reduce the sense of alienation among the group members. They validate each other's experiences but also safely challenge each other's ideas and attitudes, moving to a more objective understanding of themselves and their world. What better way to achieve such self-awareness than through association with peers in a group doing something together, the natural modality for adolescent identity formation.

Adolescents at risk yearn for something that excites them and makes them feel good. All too often they don't feel either. So much around them makes them feel lost or dead. To support a healthy self-esteem for high-risk or offender youth, they need programming that excites them and challenges them and focuses on their strengths, not on the mistakes they have made. Andrew Malekoff (2004) explains, "there is a need to tap into and honor the natural forces of youth rather than attempt to exorcise them" (p. 27). When youth feel honored and valued, they are more able to build a respectful relationship with the adult leader and fellow members, creating a safe space for growth and change. When something enters their life that wakes them up and helps them feel they belong, have a purpose and are believed in, they can finally feel that they matter.

REFERENCES

Borduin, C. and Schaeffer, C. (1998). Violent offending in adolescence: Epidemiology, correlates, outcomes and treatment. In T. Gullotta, G. Adams and R. Montemayor (Eds.), *Delinquent violent youth: Theory and interventions*. Thousand Oaks, CA: Sage, 144-174.

Brandler, S. and Roman, C. (1991). *Group work: Skills and strategies for effective interventions*. New York: The Haworth Press, Inc.

Brothers Against Guns (2004). *Final violence prevention for the San Francisco Department of Public Health*. Unpublished material.

Calhoun G., Glaser, B. and Bartolomucci, C. (2001). Counseling the juvenile offender. In A. Horne and M. Kiselica (Eds.), *Handbook of counseling boys and adolescent males*. Thousand Oaks, CA: Sage Publications, 25-34.

Carr, M. and Vandiver, T. (2001). Risk and protective factors among youth offenders. *Adolescence*, 36(143), 409-426.

Centers for Disease Control and Prevention (2005). Preventing youth violence. *Programs in Brief*. Atlanta, GA: Website.

Clark, M. (2001). Influencing positive behavior change: Increasing the therapeutic approach of juvenile courts. *Federal Probation*, 65(1), 18-27.

Cote, J. (1996). Identity: A multidimensional analysis. In G. Adams, R. Montemayor and T. Gullotta (Eds.), *Psychological development during adolescence: Progress in developmental contextualism*. Thousand Oaks, CA: Sage, 130-180.

Duffy, Trudy K. (2001). White gloves and cracked vases: How metaphors help group workers construct new perspectives and responses. *Social Work with Groups*, 24(3/4), 89-99.

Fashimpar, Gary A. (1991) From probation to mini-bikes: A comparison of traditional and innovative programs for community treatment of delinquent adolescents. *Social Work with Groups*, 14(2), 105-118.

Fatout, M., (1996). *Children in groups: A social work perspective*. Westport, CT: Greenwood Publishing.

Franz, J. (2001). Strength-based juvenile justice practice. *Wraparound and the Juvenile Justice System; Advance Practice Workshop Materials*, unpublished materials. Anaheim, CA.

Gerber, M. (1998). Winning isn't everything: A group work approach to sports teams. *Social Work with Groups*, 21(3), 35-48.

Hodge, K. and Danish, S. (2001). Promoting life skills for adolescent males through sports. In A. Horne and M. Kiselica (Eds.), *Handbook of counseling boys and adolescent males*. Thousand Oaks, CA: Sage, 55-71.

Izzo, R.L. and Ross, R.R. (1990). Meta-analysis of rehabilitation programs for juvenile delinquents: A brief report. *Criminal Justice and Behavior*, 17, 134-142.

Lerner, R. and Galambos, N. (1998). Adolescent development: Challenges, and opportunities for research, programs and policies. *Annual Review of Psychology*, 49, 413-446.

Malekoff, A. (2004). *Group work with adolescents: Principles and Practice, second edition*. New York: Guilford Press.

Malekoff, A. (1997). *Group work with adolescents: Principles and practice*. New York: Guilford Press.

Malekoff, A. (2001). The power of group work with kids: A practitioner's reflection on strengths-based practice. *Families in Society: The Journal of Contemporary Human Services*, 82(3), 243-249.

Middleman, R. and Wood, G. (1985). Maybe it's a priest or a lady with a hat with a tree on it, or is it a bumble bee?! Teaching group workers to see. *Journal of Teaching in Social Work*, 8(1/2), 129-145.

Middleman, R. and Wood, G. (1990). *Skills for direct practice in social work*. New York: Columbia University Press.

Mishna, F. and Muskat, B. (2001). Social group work for young offenders with learning disabilities. *Social Work with Groups*, 24(3/4), 11-31.

Northen, H. and Kurland, R. (2001). *Social work with groups: 3rd edition.* New York: Columbia University Press.

Osofsky, H. and Osofsky, J. (2001). Violent and aggressive behavior in youth: A mental health and prevention perspective. *Psychiatry: Interpersonal and Biological Processes,* 64(4), 285-295.

Riner, M. E. and Saywell, R. M. (2002). Development of the social ecology model of adolescent interpersonal violence prevention (SEMAIVP). *Journal of School Health,* February, 2002, Vol. 72, No. 2, 65-70.

Rose, S. (1998). *Group therapy with troubled youth: A cognitive-behavioral treatment approach.* Thousand Oaks, CA: Sage Publications.

Spielberg, W. (2001). A cultural critique of current practices of male adolescent identity formation. In A. Horne and M. Kiselica (Eds.), *Handbook of counseling boys and adolescent males.* Thousand Oaks, CA: Sage, 25-34.

Stanton, C. and Meyer A. (1998). A comprehensive review of community based approaches for the treatment of juvenile offenders. In T. Gullotta, G. Adams and R. Montemayor (Eds.), *Delinquent violent youth: Theory and interventions.* Thousand Oaks, CA: Sage, 205-229.

United States Amateur Boxing (2005). *Official rulebook and history.* Unpublished materials.

Viney, L., Truneckova, D., Weeks P. and Oades, L. (1999). Personal construct group work for adolescent offenders: Dealing with their problematic meanings. *Journal of Child and Adolescent Group Therapy,* 9(4), 187-197.

Wright, W. (1999). The use of purpose in on-going activity groups: A framework for maximizing the therapeutic impact. *Social Work with Groups,* 22(2/3), 31-54.

You Don't Always Have to Pick Up
Your Mess Right Away:
How Being Messy Can Be Really Neat!

Vicki Hallas

SUMMARY. The purpose of this paper is to illustrate a first year student's field placement experience at a group home for mentally ill adolescent boys. Upon discovering she has to "un-learn" past "learned" group work skills, she eagerly anticipates future opportunities to utilize "re-learned" theory acquired from major method course readings and lectures. Once in the field, she confronts the difficulties that this presents. The following is an account of the fears and frustrations as well as the joys and rewards one student encountered while attempting to apply and practice group work methodology in the field. *[Article copies available for a fee from The Haworth Document Delivery Service: 1-800-HAWORTH. E-mail address: <docdelivery@haworthpress.com> Website: <http://www.HaworthPress.com> © 2006 by The Haworth Press, Inc. All rights reserved.]*

KEYWORDS. Field placement, beginnings, middles, endings, supervision and survival, group home, staying in the mess, first year, relationship between facilitators, knots and groups

This article is dedicated to Sharoya Llopiz, *in memoriam*, a classmate in Roselle Kurland's group work class. Sharoya passed away in February 2005, passing on her love of life, learning, and laughter to us all.

[Haworth co-indexing entry note]: "You Don't Always Have to Pick Up Your Mess Right Away: How Being Messy Can Be Really Neat!." Hallas, Vicki. Co-published simultaneously in *Social Work with Groups* (The Haworth Press, Inc.) Vol. 29, No. 2/3, 2006, pp. 175-194; and: *Making Joyful Noise: The Art, Science, and Soul of Group Work* (ed: Andrew Malekoff, Robert Salmon, and Dominique Moyse Steinberg) The Haworth Press, Inc., 2006, pp. 175-194. Single or multiple copies of this article are available for a fee from The Haworth Document Delivery Service [1-800-HAWORTH, 9:00 a.m. - 5:00 p.m. (EST). E-mail address: docdelivery@haworthpress.com].

doi:10.1300/J009v29n02_12

INTRODUCTION: THE INTERVIEW INTERNECINE

Before I started my field work practicum, I scheduled an interview with my supervisor as a suggested protocol in order to become acquainted with her and with the agency. I soon met two supervisors instead of one, both of whom I found agreeable and friendly. After the initial exchange of pleasantries and introductions, my caseload was announced. "You'll start off slow, only three cases at first," one supervisor said as she smiled. This was followed by a lull of silence, leading me to eventually inquire about the groups. That instigated both supervisors to look at each other with some perplexity and a piece of paper with purple Hunter College letterhead being placed in front of me. It listed my name, address, and other information and functioned as a makeshift centerpiece for us to adore. "It's admirable," she began, "your interest in groups. I mean, I can't say many caseworkers would go the extra mile. Why groups?" she interrogated. "I'm a group work major," I confessed with confusion. "You are?" gasped the other supervisor. "But your field assignment says casework. See, right here," she pointed to the sheet of paper–our centerpiece. My name was printed clearly in bold and caps. Next to it were the two letters "G" and "W," also in bold caps. Not knowing really what to say I attempted to clarify the confusion nicely. I cleared my throat and proposed, "I believe GW means group work." Another lull of silence as one supervisor uttered in disbelief, "GW? GW! But we haven't ever had a group work student before!" She ogled her co-worker and snatched the piece of paper scrambling to decipher the enigmatic code. Brooding for a little, she eventually concluded aloud: "You're right! It says GW. I'll call your advisor to confirm." Then, as she hesitated . . . "I'm not sure I supervise group workers." The other supervisor interjected, "Why not? We have a ton of groups." Releasing a somewhat painful noise, the other supervisor sighed, "You're right. Lord knows we have groups galore!" They laughed together. Then they both smiled and looked at me with pity as if to say, *forgive her Father for she knows not what she says.* I left the interview without any discussion of the "groups galore." Was this a bad sign?

Days later at Hunter our advisors met with their students. We went around the room and introduced ourselves. It was the usual drill: name, field placement, major method. I was the last to go and finished my sentence with a boastful smile, "major method: group work." My advisor nodded at me and then stopped midway, baffled. "Group Work? I don't have any group work advisees. Are you sure?" she asked? "I think you might have one now," I grinned, hopeful. I was beginning to feel like a character in a Kafka movie. I wondered when this same scene would cease to replay itself or if it would just continue to play over and over again. *Please make it stop* (fade to black . . .).

Bewildered, my advisor rummaged through her bag and displayed a piece of paper with the same purple letterhead: the all-too-familiar makeshift centerpiece. "Your advisement sheet says casework. You changed your method already?" The other students began to chuckle. "Who wants to do group work?" one student hollered. "I know," added another. "It's so much work and no reward . . . so NOT worth it, ya know?" rolling her eyes as the other students all sat colluding in the joke with a nod here and a moan there.

My advisor dragged the sheet of paper over to where I was sitting and pointed to the letters printed in bold and caps next to my name. "See here," she said slowly, "it states CW. That's for casework: C-A-S-E-W-O-R-K," she crooned. *Here we go again!* "Actually," I corrected her, nonplused, "it says G-W. That's for group work." My advisor then strategically placed the paper up to the light in an attempt to decipher the faded "GW" palimpsest, a riddle wrapped in a puzzle. Examining the enigma with more scrutiny she jolted, "You're right!" *Eureka,* I thought. "I've never had a group work student before," she chimed in astonishment. "If it makes you feel any better," she said sympathetically, "you're at the right place. Hunter's *the place* for group work," she preened.

At this point, besides my annoyance I felt anger. Yet, I also felt motivated. Somehow this double misreading of text in the form of two large initials gave me the impetus to start reading the literature assigned to us in class and to use my log, a tabula rasa soon to be seething with scathing scribble in script. It is apropos, therefore, that I began judging the articles by their cover and selected the last article first solely based on its title, "Caught in the Doorway Between Education and Practice: Group Work's Battle For Survival" (Kurland and Salmon, 2002).

And so this is how it all began: starting my first log entry with the last article in the course pack–my modus operandi. The article uses Shakespeare's King Henry the Fifth as an example of group workers who struggle to win an arduous battle against a casework-centered profession (see also Kurland and Salmon, 1996). Like King Henry, I felt galvanized by the armada of French invaders. I too, was dodging for cover, outraged by the blitzkrieg of "CW" napalm and shrapnel. After reading more about the history and plight of group work, however (see, for example, Middleman, 1990; and Tropp, 1978), I was encouraged. I too wanted to rally my group work troops. In my mind, I gathered the necessary war accoutrements in preparation, shouting out at my comrades from under the garrison running into battle heralding, "Once more unto the breach dear friends, once more; or close the wall up with our English dead!" (Kurland and Salmon, 2002, p. 1). I was ready to ward off the enemy who misread a "GW" as a "CW." How dare they! *Et tu, Brutus*? Willing to fight to the death against every last barbarian invasion who saw a "C" instead of a "G" I would rise to the occasion from underneath the bivouac battling CW reconnaissance! I mustered in the name of a "GW" NOT a "CW," "once more unto the breach, dear friends . . ." (Kurland and Salmon, 2002, p. 14).

FIELD PLACEMENT: FANTASY OR FALLACY?

It was the first day of field placement, and my assignment included interning at three different group homes for adolescents and an alternative high school in Westchester County, New York. My supervisor and I were driving from one group home to the other in her car, and I was about to meet the second set of teenage boys (16-21) who resided at this particular home. The drive was about twenty minutes, and being accustomed to the city I felt as if I was headed to a Bed & Breakfast in the country for the weekend. The roads twisted ever further upward past the Hudson River revealing one more gorgeous mansion after another. Endless rows of trees bursted with branch tips budding leaves to tickle roof tops as the wind exhaled her breath. Dawn would soon surrender to dusk, and dusk would soon slip and fall into night. It was the kind of day when the sky simmers in warm hues of golds, reds, and purples. I looked out the window and noticed the Palisades cascading downward into the reflection of the clouds rippling on top of the river. *Is this a dream? Did Hunter make some sort of mistake?*

At the top of a hill in the midst of a wooded and affluent residential area, my supervisor slowed down, pulled her car over to park, and smiled at me. "We're here," she said. As if standing while asleep an old blue Victorian home leaned to the left. Graciously corpulent, Old Victoria was a stunning somnambulant. Her enormous oval windows blinked awake taking in a glance of me, giving me a once-over. "The eyes are the windows of the soul," I recalled not fully appreciating the Edgar Allan Poe reference at that moment. "You'll not be welcome here," my supervisor hissed. "You'll be looked upon with suspicion and skepticism," she whispered. Dread soon filled my body. As we hiked up the steep staircase, I noticed a young boy of about sixteen talking rapidly into the air and swatting something he thought was flying around him. My supervisor scoffed, "that's a resident. He's lived here for over four years. He hears voices and sees things. He's crazy. Many of them are crazy here. Quick!" she spat loudly bolting toward the front door. Suddenly, the estate I once revered with awe transformed into a dilapidated, haunted house. I started to become afraid. Was that a noise? Did I just hear a wolf howl? Oh my god! It's the falling "House of Usher!" (I should not have mentioned Edgar Allan Poe!)

In fact, my experience with the residents at this group home was anything but unwelcome even though it is completely appropriate for adolescents who have been abused by their parents to look at strangers with some suspicion–almost a survival skill. Most "healthy" adolescents do not openly embrace and accept any stranger–let alone an adult *slash* student *slash* intern who is to study them in "their own home." This was not even Beginnings according to prudent stage development, so they were supposed to hesitate (Garland et al., 1973). It is uncanny when professionals who claim to be experts at working with adolescents seem to be the same individuals who know the least about this very population they are working with or seem to make the effort to understand the complex challenges and vicissitudes of adolescence.

Nonetheless, afternoon soon became evening, and I gladly accepted the invitation to eat dinner with the kids. Dinner consisted of the usual appetizer: *scanning*, followed by the popular entrée: *discomfort*. Later served a familiar palate cleanser: *risk-taking*, and finally, saving room for the best, dessert arrived: *humor*.

As my field placement proceeded, I learned this particular group home had been in existence for over fifteen years without ever having one group for residents! A group home that never had groups–the quintessential oxymoron. The social worker with whom I would co-facilitate three groups was a new hire; she had started two months prior and suggested groups on her second day. Her suggestion had been met with skepticism and suspicion, the same that I had been warned about by administration regarding the clients. Criticized for wanting to incorporate groups she was viewed as "lazy" for not wanting to do "real work" and questioned *ad nauseum* about the reason for groups in the first place. "Thank god you're a group worker" she said, exasperated. "Because of you I can finally run groups! If I want to run groups people act like I'm blowing off work, but if I supervise you then I'm seen as working!" Informed in my group work class to expect this type of response, I had heard group workers were viewed in the field as people who cannot or do not want to do "serious clinical work." Now my third supervisor (not that I was counting!) continued. "No one thinks running groups is therapy. They actually think its down time. Of course, they're harder to do than individual work, which is why no one wants to do them," she added, becoming red in the face. I noticed a hint of perspiration on her forehead as she stopped to pour herself some water. She concluded, "I'm just glad you're here."

Honestly? I could not actually say the same. At this point I was very worried and did not want to be supervised by someone who did not study group work. Did she just say "run groups" instead of working "with" or "within" groups? (Middleman and Wood, 1990). A passage from a recent reading emerged: "Practitioners from other disciplines and group 'facilitators' often say they *run* groups. When they speak of working with individuals they do not speak of running individuals! Yet they run groups. Such a curious vocabulary says something about subtle, professional-technical, elitist orientations, and thus about the control issues involved in treating or facilitating groups" (Middleman and Wood, 1990, p. 91). One thought could not escape me: how does a group home for adolescent boys not have groups–not even groups that are *run*?

GROUPS GALORE!

Shortly thereafter I was assigned to co-facilitate a total of six groups: three pre-established ones at one site already using group work and three new ones at that residential facility. They only came with titles, however, indicating gender and time of day, which was obfuscating and vastly general. "When a group's purpose is stated at a high level of generality, it has little meaning to its members" (Northen and Kurland, 2001, p. 177). With much chagrin, I perused the group titles I was to *work with*:

1. Girls Morning Group
2. Boys Morning Group
3. Girls Afternoon Group
4. Boys Afternoon Group (with Pizza)
5. Boys Afternoon Group (without Pizza)
6. Crazy Mom Group (for boys)

Thus, groups galore became groups *du jour*. Making assumptions is a well-known danger, but assume I did. I assumed these references were a mistake. Was it the *sans* pizza and *avec* pizza that bothered me the most? Unsure but perturbed I thought about the importance of pre-group screening, planning, and attention to group purpose. And then I got angry again and confused as well. It was crucial to know what I was doing, but in fact, I had no clue and neither did anyone else, apparently. I recalled what I read some time before, "knowing what they are going to do is not enough. Members need to understand why they are doing it" (Northen and Kurland, 2001, p. 176). So not only did the members not understand what they were doing or why, neither did the facilitators! (I included myself in the facilitator category and realized this was an egregious example of the "All-in-the-Same-Boat" Phenomenon (Shulman, 1999).)

Could it get any worse? No, I thought. But it did. I observed three such "groups" at the school site and became immediately traumatized. Starting to show signs of survivor guilt just from bearing witness to these so-called groups, I began to see why none of the adolescents wanted to attend them. First, they were on group overload, because the program mandated two groups per day, five days a week. Second, what they were there for (purpose) and what they should do (content) were nebulous and mercurial. So I started to spend some time hanging out with them, and eventually I gained a better understanding of their needs and interests (Malekoff, 2004). I reached for my Tylenol and sought out my supervisor.

SOMETIMES BEING MESSY CAN BE REALLY NEAT

My supervisor began with an informative lesson: it was common knowledge among professionals in the social work field that those who were refused by Hunter the first time around applied for group work on their second go-round, guaranteed admission: *the expert*. She then elaborated on her aversion to loud groups: *the kill joy*. She cringed at loud disruptive groups: *the prima donna*. Loud groups inferred a lacked of discipline, she said: *the judge* . . . "I just won't have it!" *the bully*. "If the group lacked discipline, the group leader lacked discipline": *the intellectual*. Her disdain for the type of group work so many of us should do resonated in the class literature, "group work with kids is rarely neat" (Malekoff, 2004, p. 19).

Group workers often find themselves disrespected in the field because of the raucous and mess group work permits and enjoys: *the troublemaker*. This is reverberated in a common group work bind, "we get no respect because our groups make noise and move about, vibrate and explode, laugh and have fun. But all this does not happen by accident even though, at times, group workers are ashamed and apologetic. 'Sorry,' they say, "next time I'll try to keep them more quiet . . . from making such a mess . . . from leaving the room," (Malekoff, 2004, p. 19).

The disdain toward groups that my supervisor displayed directly contradicted some of the best lectures I had heard delineating group work techniques, such as, "don't rush to solutions" and "stay in the mess." So while I learned to "stay in the mess" as a student, as an intern, I was told not to make one. As a student I learned that being messy meant building courage and strengthening skills, but as an intern I learned that being messy meant simply picking up the mess you should have never made in the first place.

So, what is a "mess," exactly? *The Random House Dictionary* (1966, p. 899) defines mess, this noun *thoust vexes,* in interesting priority: definition number one is rudimentary: "dirty or untidy." Definition number two is an "embarrassing confusion." (Ironically, confusion resonates for group workers because it is seen as opportunity for change, growth, and even cohesion.) Definition numbers five to eight may raise some eyebrows in their linkage of "mess" to an action that a collective group of people share: "5. a group regularly taking meals together. 6. the meal so taken. 7. See mess hall. 8. Naval. Messroom." After number 10, more disturbing pictures become "mess" is sketched: "12: Informal. a person whose life or affairs are in a state of confusion, esp. a person with a confused or disorganized moral or psychological outlook." Finally, the penultimate definition could jolt any group worker with its mere use of familiar semantic, "18. mess around or about, a. *Informal.* to busy oneself without purpose or plan; work half-heartedly; putter. b. *Slang.* to waste time; loaf. c. *Slang.* to involve or associate (oneself) with, esp. for informal or unethical purposes . . ."

In brief, what is a mess to one is not necessarily a mess for others! In group work messy means serious about the work and "thinking group" (Kurland and Salmon, 1992; Middleman and Wood, 1990). Life is messy; and groups are like life. Intimacy is messy, and groups are intimate. Does that mean life is a disheveled "waste of time?" Is intimacy just another sloppy "unethical loafer?" Is life lived only by a bunch of "half-hearted putters?" In the end this plethora of definitions did offer three cogent tenets: groups need a purpose: *the ally* (Northen and Kurland, 2001). Group workers need to plan: *a key activity* (Northen and Kurland, 2001, p.110). And group workers need to be ethical.

In groups, the messy ebb of intimacy often intersects with life flow as portrayed in Deborah Luepintz's work, *Schopenhauer's Porcupines* (2002). Curiously, Schopenhauer's fable about porcupines is cited by Freud in one of his books on group psychology (Luepintz, 2002). Luepintz, who illustrates the discomfort and intimacy that porcupines share in their life cycle, touches upon one of the most important nuances in the "middle" stage of group development and coincidentally speaks to the need of "staying in the mess" that so many workers desire.

Once, when Luepintz was on a private tour of Freud's London home, the author took note of a small porcupine statue, drawing upon Schopenhauer's porcupine fable with her tour guide (2002):

> A troop of porcupines is milling about on a cold winter's day. In order to keep from freezing, the animals move closer together. Just as they are close enough to huddle, however, they start to poke each other with their quills. In order to stop the pain, they spread out, lose the advantage of commingling, and again begin to shiver. This sends them back in search of each other, and the cycle repeats as they struggle to find a comfortable distance between entanglement and freezing. (p. 2)

Like the freezing porcupines who come together for warmth, groups too come together. Some members poke at each other with their quills: *conflict*. At times, this may be a misunderstanding: *trust*. Occasionally, it may be rather deliberate: *opposing defenses*. Members may attempt to get closer to one another in an effort to escape the cold: *need*. They may depend on the warmth of others: *vulnerability*. Some may verbalize it out loud: *taking risks*. Others may reciprocate this same need for warmth: *mutual aid*. At times, no one may agree: *differences in opinion*. This may lead to tension: *confrontation*. That may result in a fight: *crisis*. A few may retreat and distance: *isolating*. But several may come together: *intimacy*.

In fact, all of these circumstances involve a level of intimacy, trust, and risk: *human interaction*, feelings that can be trying, entangling, and messy: *group cohesion*.

Similar to the porcupines, group members struggle to find comfort and safety as they huddle and spread out: *resolutions*. Of course, comfort and safety take time: *don't rush to solutions*. But it is that struggle, encompassed in a mess of fear and discomfort, that a stand-up kind of group worker plans for, what we group workers are trained to face, what we hope, in fact, will happen, because it is the heart and soul of the work–our work: group work.

If group members are forbidden to have "messy" feelings and instead encouraged to have "neat" feelings, group process is not only compromised as "squeeky clean," it is annihilated and made obsolete; and demands that the worker "learn to move in and feel, then move out and process, all the while staying with feelings" seems applicable under this tutelage (Roman, 2002, p. 62). Teaching a student instrumental skills needed when members are "entangled" or "freezing," such as reaching for, getting with, and staying with feelings, becomes thwarted if agencies dictate definitions of "acceptable" emotions (Middleman and Wood, 1990). The first year can be a fruitful one, therefore, as students learn from others how to tolerate the "chaos and not (get) pulled into it" (Roman, 2002, p. 62); but it can also be a disenchanting one if students never see the fruits of their labor. As interns we may teeter across the rope that dangles above the precipice without a net, floundering as the field work funambulist; and often during that first year of mine I wondered if it would not be easier to remain reticent like so many others: *an established norm?*

Staying within feelings insinuates that "staying in the mess" is vital to mutual aid (Steinberg, 2004)–an essential apparatus for healing, a conduit to comprehensive care and a sacrosanct service in applying theory to practice. Like porcupines, life and groups can be prickly, and we may get poked. Like life, groups can be messy, and we may be a mess. But sometimes, being messy is really neat, because it is *group work.*

THE SUPERVISION OF SISYPHUS

Often toward the end of supervision I would feel as if my fate was an eternal punishment: *the victim* (a repetitive uphill battle with baggage: *the rock*); and on more than one occasion I "jumped to solutions" in order to escape the torturous tête-à-tête trek. For example, in response to the list of group titles, I suggested we substitute activity-based groups, such as a reading group for the mentally ill boys, a knitting group for girls, and an additional drama-therapy group for girls who bully. I wanted groups with purpose; furthermore, I wanted to address the huge number of groups in which the teenagers had to participate. Particularly disconcerting was the dilemma that a group home with little to no group history now mandated residents to three per week! I feared the "over-group"conundrum and wanted to toss a rope overboard (I did not even mention or address the "crazy mom" group!). In short, I could not muster the necessary patience at this point, so I capitulated: *the Polyanna, the saint, the ingenue, the teacher's pet*; and so the outcome of the planning meeting was predictable:

1. Friday afternoon groups must have pizza.
2. No bully groups.
3. No budget allotment for needles or yarn (needles were a concern).
4. All books must be approved prior to the group's first meeting.
5. All books approved must be read.
6. Do not expect "these types of clients to actually read."
7. Every member of the group must speak, at least once, in every group.

Fortunately, the meeting was not a *total knockout*. I took a few good hits, some even below the belt, as it were (since everyone must be allowed to speak) and some at the jugular (everyone must be allowed to speak in every group). I was told that I needed to understand the population (i.e., no one will be able to read): *Round One*. I sparred and was still standing: *Round Two*. Black and blue, I lost the knitting group, but forever the pugilist I held onto the ropes: *Round Three*. I came out of the corner back into the ring (I'll ask for the knitting group again): *Round Four*. But someone had to stitch me up (no bully groups): *Round Five*. The first group would be the reading group scheduled to meet the next day in the field: *Round Six*. I was down, but not out (I got a reading group). I didn't throw in the towel. *The thrill of victory; the agony of defeat–a moral victory.*

The reading group was comprised of five randomly selected boys: *composition predetermined*. There was no pre-group contact, no screening, and no planning. *Mea culpa!* I learned that most of the members suffer from a learning disorder or attention deficit disorder; that all except one maintained excellent attendance, enjoyed most classes, and liked reading (most things); were motivated to study and worried about grades (except one). The only overall complaint I heard about was the lack of quiet time or study time after chores. Finally, from hanging out I learned there was a need to read (Malekoff, 2004).

I SEE YOUR MIDDLES AND CHALLENGE YOU TO BEGINNINGS

Although I was in Beginnings with the group and it was in Beginnings with itself, the members were in Middles with each other (Garland et al.,

1973), tainting my initial feeling about the group's Beginnings. Group workers in residential settings may commonly experience members who live together as roommates but do not know one another as co-members of a group. When this happens, the Beginning stage swings pendulously to and fro toward Middles and back again, challenging the worker and the whole system. In response, I decided to focus on the nearsightedness of the group and zoomed in on the group's here and now: we were all in Beginnings as a group even though the members were in Middles with one another. This vision was blurry, and I referred to my myopia as the "Bringing it Back to Beginnings" Phenomenon.

Since I was the latest addition to the group, I became a bit nervous. All of the group members had lived together for at least one year; three of the members had lived in the group home together for a total of four years; and their level of comfort with each other was high. My level of comfort, in contrast, was low, a dynamic that augmented my anxiety in some ways but truncated it in others. After all, many Beginning-stage difficulties that facilitators encounter may be assuaged if group members already know one other. For example, inviting full participation, reaching for a feeling link, and building on strengths were all easier in this group than usual (Middleman and Wood, 1990). Communication among the adolescents flowed even if I did not: *sleuth out information.* Each member offered a wealth of information about the others; behaviors, strengths, and weaknesses were discussed openly and with much detail. Members prided themselves on knowing one another's pet-peeves and idiosyncrasies.

While familiarity may offer an expedited level of comfort and intimacy, it is also true that it might oscillate into exacerbated conflict. Since these group members knew one another, however, they concentrated on me so that scanning, verbalizing norms, and referring to purpose presented more of a challenge (Middleman and Wood, 1990). In fact, during one of my attempts to scan a group member yelled out, "Why are you doing that thing with your neck again?" Looking at the others, he added, "What's her deal?" Another time while I was trying to establish rules one member asked, "Are you a teacher or something? I think you left your ruler outside!"

Of course, I know that planning would have mitigated much of this distress (Northen and Kurland, 2001), but planning never did take place, as the facilitator was swamped with meetings. "No one understands the significance of planning a group," she huffed. "I've been up to my neck in meetings–sorry," she apologized only to then leave the group three times to answer her cell phone. "It's an emergency," she apologized each time.

Seemingly, establishing group norms was difficult; members were accustomed to the "way things were," so that when I tried to establish new norms I was met with "Naaahuh, we can so eat . . . that's not a rule!" and "Yaaahuh, we can so interrupt . . . we always do!"

Agency culture has its own set of rules and norms, rules and norms that may conflict with group culture, which also has a set of rules and norms. When the two collide "the agency's structure, policies, and procedures" often "influence matters of access, continuity, equity, and quality of services" (Northen and Kurland, 2001, p. 115). Staff and agencies may feel threatened or burdened by group presence and its mores (see Malekoff, 2004); and staff may have to consider, even if inconvenient, a change in procedures (Northen and Kurland, 2001). One such example occurred during an early group meeting. Members were introducing themselves when the door was kicked open with tremendous force. Ricocheting against the wall, it caused a loud "bang" followed by a huge "thud" and two child care workers hurtling into the room, screaming and laughing. As members whizzed their heads around the room completely startled, one employee rigorously snapped a camera while the other employee shouted, "GROUP PHOTO!" The two left as quickly as they arrived, while we remained stunned and blinded by the flash.

Concomitantly, I thought about Beginnings in relation to location. When the group meets in the members' home, such as a residential facility, the usual level of early discomfort related to Beginnings may lessen; at the same time, it may bring forth an increase in "acting-out" behavior or "authority testing" (Northen and Kurland, 2001). Ultimately, in this group certain facets of Beginnings and Middles actually coalesced smoothly, with group members appearing well adjusted and relaxed without stress from traveling to the meeting or adjusting to a new context or environment. In effect, the transition was mitigated at this point rather than exacerbated because of common ground, although I couldn't say as much for the staff.

Critical to Beginnings is the relationship between co-facilitators. In this first session, the facilitator was astoundingly affable and respectful, using language to indicate the importance of my role and of my value to the group and agency, and helping the group to feel a certain level of trust and assurance. Her affinity for my presence encouraged a sense of safety otherwise strenuous to attain (Wright, 2002).

A good rapport between facilitators is paramount, and I cannot emphasize its value to the group. Co-facilitating with someone who is distant, vituperative, or incendiary can so easily result in a tumultuous and disheartening experience for all (Wright, 2002). Profound emphasis should be placed on the relationship between facilitators, therefore, as it exudes into the group dynamic instigating possible distress. Traces of this unfortunate predicament, fortunately, did not enter into our relationship (during this session or throughout the entire year). Even though she had a penchant for missing Planning and Purpose meetings, I remained cognizant and appreciative of her myriad, other redeeming qualities.

Toward the end of this first group, the goal was announced by the facilitator: to create a list of three books the group would like to read. We would order the books so everyone could have their own and keep them in the group room so they would not get "misplaced" as things often "were." Rules were never concretely established at this point except for a verbatim amalgam of jokes and preferences:

1. No farting because it made the room smell, "and you know that means you, Jerald."
2. No burping because it caused competition between group members resulting in uncontrollable, never-ending burp contests, "and you know that means you Jerald and Mark!" (Apparently, they shared a jaded past of competing for attention.)
3. No sleeping because it was "wack" and "some people don't know how to act thinking they are in the Bronx Zoo! And that means you Mark, so don't lie about it and be a hater!"

A new rule was added:

4. No interruptions during group from staff "and that goes for photos during group especially if it's Robert or Al because they are so annoying!"

The members expressed excitement about a reading group and voted on the books making a list:

1. *Malcolm X.*
2. Poems by Maya Angelou (two members had mothers who loved Maya Angelou).
3. Shakespeare's *The Tragedy of Othello* (two members had to read it for class).

4. Any book on animals (wild animals and not household, domesticated pets. The notion was conveyed that pets were restricted and not allowed to do anything fun).
5. *The Color Purple* by Alice Walker (the two members who said their moms loved Maya Angelou said their moms also loved Oprah Winfrey).
6. Any book on Madrid (three group members had a paper to do on Spain).

The next topic quickly moved on to "rewards." The group expressed a desire to be rewarded for reading. "Reading books is hard, so we deserve a reward," yelled Jerald. The rest of the group agreed. A list was then compiled which prioritized rewards in this order:

1. Seeing a movie on the book.
2. Seeing a movie on the author if there were no movies on a poem.
3. Seeing a movie on the animals the book was about.
4. Seeing a movie on the city or country the book was about.
5. Seeing the most recent movie on the book "not a boring old one like the played-out version of *Othello* with Laurence Fishburne, who is old school . . . cuz the movie O with Mekhi Phifer is all-that!"
6. Eating foods from different countries the books talk about. For example, eating food from Spain or going out to a Spanish restaurant, "and that doesn't mean Taco Bell. Because Taco Bell is Mexican."
7. "Movies have to have not just pizza either but popcorn, too."

"IF THIS IS WEEK FOUR, WE MUST BE DOING READING?"

Not only were we not reading at this point, we didn't have the books. Not only did we not have the books, the books hadn't been ordered. Not only were the books not ordered, the books hadn't been approved . . .

I pressed my supervisor to approve a book from the list we submitted, so we could order members their own individualized copies (flummoxed, I fretted over whether or not the library would have five copies of the same book). "Maybe we should examine your need for a security blanket," my supervisor slithered out. "I'm sorry?" I began. "What is it about external, physical gadgets that make you feel better prepared as a clinician?" she pined. "It's a reading group? We sort of need the books in order to read? You wanted to approve the books before we ordered them?" I stared blankly hoping it would pass for *looking with planned emptiness* (Middleman and Wood, 1990). In one of our class lectures, Professor Kurland discussed a group work student who was in Middles with a cooking group. I related to the part of the story when the kitchen ovens broke and remained broken until Endings. The worker baked the cakes at home and brought them in for the group to eat. I should just buy five copies of *Malcolm* X. Will my credit card go through? My supervisor concluded, "you'll read *Harry Potter*. Go ahead and order five of them." *Harry Potter? The coup de grâce.*

TO KNOT OR NOT TO KNOT?
TIS THE QUESTION OF CONCLUSIONS

The group waited for *Harry Potter* with unforeseen poise and elan; meantime, they decided to read from either a homework assignment, a journal entry (three members were journaling) or a collected "favorite pick" of the week (a show-and-tell reading to discuss). One particular group will always stand out in my mind with fond tenderness because of no particular one reason. In all honesty, it was the kind of group that should have stood out in my mind for all the many wrong reasons. It was memorable not because of the succinct and comprehensive implementation of Context, Planning, Purpose, Composition, Structure, Content, Screening or Pre-Group Contact. But there was Need (*sotto voce*)? There was a need for the members to have a relationship with one another and with themselves in a room of their own where they could think and talk with direction and without demand (duty calls in chores) or disruption (*non sequitur* noise). At one point I thought about Chapter Three of Northen and Kurland (2001) titled, "Relationships: The Heart of Practice" and its comparison: "a group is a 'relationship laboratory'" (p. 73). I knew this laboratory space was not nearly enough, but the bunsen burners kindled a small flame-simmering connection. It demonstrated how "people need people; they are social organisms from birth on" (2001, p. 55). Still, even though it was the oft-described anti-group situation it was still somehow a start with soupçon of steadiness and a partial wholeness. "The whole is determined, not only by its constituents, but also by the relationship of the parts to one another and to the environment"(2001, p. 35). It was as if the old relationships in this new laboratory created a reborn rhythm. A murmur of melody gestated sounding from underneath the usual unharmonious cacophony of communication. It was the quintessential first-year student's must "un-learn" and then "re-learn" group. Yet, it was the kind of group so many first years end up doing and re-doing. I felt a sense of chagrin for feeling a sense of pride as a moment in time ticked toward the group interacting with one another honestly and fully. "People's lives are enriched when the need for a strong human connection is met–one that is accepting, genuine, and empathetic" (Northen and Kurland, 2001, p. 55). And it was wonderful to sit in it all–to sit *within* and *with* its everything–the beauty of empathy and the beast of acceptance. *It was a mess!*

As group was about to begin, one member picked up a xerox copy of a poem from my desk: *Knots,* by R.D. Laing. I had copied it after Professor Kurland read it to our class, intending to frame it for my office. The group started tossing it around the room making fun of the fact that I had homework, yelling in unison, "Vic's pics!" After much persuasion and pressure, they voted on reading my presumed "homework." Each member took turns reading out loud (p. 56).

There is something I don't know
that I am supposed to know. *(laughter)*
I don't know *what* it is I don't know,
and yet am supposed to know, *(laughter)*
and I feel I look stupid
if I seem both not to know it
and not know what it is I don't know. *(grunts of confusion)*
Therefore I pretend I know it. (silence)
This is nerve-wracking *(more grunts)*
since I don't know what I must pretend to know. *(nods in agreement)*
Therefore I pretend to know everything. *(laughter)*
I feel you know what I am supposed to know *(laughter)*
but you can't tell me what it is *(silence)*
because you don't know that I don't know what it is.
You may know what I don't know, but not *(more nods in agreement)*
that I don't know it,
and I can't tell you.
So you will have to tell me everything.

(From *Knots* by R.D. Laing, © 1970. Used by permission of Pantheon Books, a division of Random House, Inc.)

Some members read with ease while other members displayed difficulty. Some members flustered and repeated lines while others read smoothly. Each member helped out the other. A few laughed, others became confused and most nodded. Here is a snippet of the ensuing interaction:

Carl: Boy that guy's stupid! Jesus! I feel bad for him!
Jerald: You think everyone is stupid! I feel bad for you!
Mark: He's just confused is all.
Tommy: I'm confused a lot.
Jerald: Me too. I'm confused and feel stupid for being confused.
Mark: Being confused isn't being stupid.
Carl: If you're confused you look stupid.
Jerald: Only to stupid people.
Carl: My dad called me stupid.
Tommy: My mom acted like she knew it all.
Jerald: I pretend to know it all and I'm really confused. I don't want
    to look stupid.
Tommy: If you pretend to know it all people think you do.
Jerald: But you really don't.
George: I'm confused. (*laughter*)
Carl: My dad left my mom cuz she was stupid. He's stupid.
Jerald: My brother calls me stupid. He's a jerk.
Carl: If you're confused people think you're stupid. You get left behind.
    Forgotten.
Mark: I got left behind in school.
Carl: Not in school, in life . . . like, people leave you, so you should
    pretend.
Jerald: (*To Carl*) I don't think you're stupid.
George: (*To Carl*) Me neither. (*Takes candy out of his bag and puts it
    on Carl's desk*)

I gave Laing's poem, *Knots,* and the group more thought. Knots are a nuisance. I remembered the knots on my running shoes. They make me late. They annoy me. I have to spend time and patience getting them out. Time I don't have early in the morning before a run. Which string to pull out first? Should I tug at this one? Or yank at that one? The string that looks the easiest can be the hardest. The string that looks the hardest can be the easiest. Ones you have never even seen before pop up out of nowhere. After a while, you just work around it. You forget the knot was such a hassle. You adjust to it. You accept it. And expect it. I get used to slipping on my shoes and not having to bend down and tie them. The knots make it easier for me. They end up saving me time. They become part of the shoe. I appreciate them.

I thought about how knots are like groups. All bunched-up and connected together or entangled in a mesh. You try to take them apart. This is a struggle. It takes time, patience and skill to figure out. You have to use care in working with them. You have to figure out which member can be untied and when. Maybe he needs to be tugged a little? Maybe she should be pulled a bit? You have to think about the one member who isn't part of the knot. They pop up, the biggest knot of all. Maybe certain knots are better left alone. Some knots should be tightened so they won't come undone. So we won't trip and fall. Certain members shouldn't be untied at all but tightened. Members can be appreciated and accepted for the knots they offer. The group can work around their knot. Their knot can make group easier. Some group members are helpful and others are a hassle. Some are both—each offering something different. All of them can be appreciated. They make it easier for us. Ultimately, it depends on the knot and who is wearing the shoe.

REFERENCES

Bernstein, S. (1973). Conflict and group work. *Explorations in group work*. Boston: Milford House, Inc., 54-80.

Caplan, T. and Thomas, H. (2003). If this is week three, we must be doing "feelings": An essay on the importance of client-paced group work. *Social Work with Groups*, 26(3), 5-15.

Garland, J., Jones, H., and Kolodny, R. (1973). A model for stages in development in social work with groups, in S. Bernstein (Ed.), *Explorations in group work*. Boston: Milford House, 17-71.

Garvin, C., Gutierrez, L., and Galinsky, M. (2004). *Handbook of social work with groups*. New York: Guilford Press.

Kurland, R. and Salmon, R. (2002). Caught in the doorway between education and practice: Group work's battle for survival, Plenary Presentation at Symposium XXIV of the Association for the Advancement of Social Work With Groups. Also in press: Cohen, C., Phillips, M., and Hanson, M., *Think group: Strength and diversity in group work*. Binghamton, NY: The Haworth Press, Inc.

Kurland, R. and Salmon, R. (1998). *Teaching a methods course in social work with groups*. Alexandria, VA: Council on the Social Work Education.

Kurland, R. and Salmon, R. (1996). Making joyful noise: Presenting, promoting and portraying group work to and for the profession, in B. Stempler and M. Glass (Eds.),

Social group work today and tomorrow: Moving from theory to advanced training and practice. Binghamton, NY: The Haworth Press, Inc., 19-32.

Kurland, R. and Salmon, R. (1993). Not just one of the gang: Group workers and their role as an authority, in P. Ephross and T. Vassil (Eds.), *Social work with groups: Expanding horizons.* Binghamton, NY: The Haworth Press, Inc., 153-169.

Laing, R.D. (1970). *Knots.* New York, NY: Random House, Inc.

Luepnitz, D. (2002). *Schopenhauer's porcupines.* New York, NY: Basic Books.

Malekoff, A. (2004). *Group work with adolescents* (2nd ed.). New York, NY: Guilford Press.

Middleman, R. (1990). Group work and the Heimlich maneuver: Unchoking social work education, in D. Fike and B. Rittner (Eds), *Working from strengths: The essence of group work.* Miami Shores, FL: Center For Group Work Studies, 16-40.

Middleman, R. and Wood, G. (1990). *Skills for direct practice in social work.* New York, NY: Columbia University Press.

Northen, H. and Kurland, R. (2001). *Social work with groups.* (3rd ed.). New York, NY: Columbia University Press.

Roberts, R. and Northen, H. (1976). Eds., *Theories of social work with groups.* New York, NY: Columbia University Press.

Roman, C. (2002). It is not always easy to sit on your mouth, in R. Kurland and A. Malekoff (Eds.), *Stories celebrating group work. It's not always easy to sit on your mouth.* Binghamton, NY: The Haworth Press, Inc., 61-64.

Shulman, L. (1999). *The skills of helping individuals, families, groups and communities* (4th ed.). Belmont, CA: Wadsworth/Thomson Learning.

Steinberg, D. (2004). *The mutual-aid approach to working with groups: Helping people help one another.* Binghamton, NY: The Haworth Press, Inc.

Tropp, E. (1978). Whatever happened to group work? *Social Work with Groups,* 1(1), 84-95.

Wright, M. (2002). Co-facilitation: Fashion or function? *Social Work with Groups,* 25(4), 77-92.

Group Work Gets Physical:
Self-Defense Class and Social Work

Sarah Stevenson

SUMMARY. This article examines how a self-defense class is a social work group when it incorporates basic group work principles. The ways in which stages of group development, member roles and mutual aid are used in a self-defense class will be explored. The article also highlights how a self-defense class can be a legitimate intervention for women who have been victimized. *[Article copies available for a fee from The Haworth Document Delivery Service: 1-800-HAWORTH. E-mail address: <docdelivery@ haworthpress.com> Website: <http://www.HaworthPress.com> © 2006 by The Haworth Press, Inc. All rights reserved.]*

KEYWORDS. Self-defense, adrenalized state, stages of group development, member roles, mutual aid

BACKGROUND

A social work group is most clearly defined as one in which personal growth and social objectives are equally emphasized. As Newstetter (1935) explained, "Group work can be defined as an educational process emphasizing (1) the development and social adjustment of an individual through voluntary group association; and (2) the use of this

[Haworth co-indexing entry note]: "Group Work Gets Physical: Self-Defense Class and Social Work." Stevenson, Sarah. Co-published simultaneously in *Social Work with Groups* (The Haworth Press, Inc.) Vol. 29, No. 2/3, 2006, pp. 195-215; and: *Making Joyful Noise: The Art, Science, and Soul of Group Work* (ed: Andrew Malekoff, Robert Salmon, and Dominique Moyse Steinberg) The Haworth Press, Inc., 2006, pp. 195-215. Single or multiple copies of this article are available for a fee from The Haworth Document Delivery Service [1-800-HAWORTH, 9:00 a.m. - 5:00 p.m. (EST). E-mail address: docdelivery@haworthpress.com].

association as a means of furthering other socially desirable ends. It is concerned therefore with both individual growth and social results. Moreover, it is the combined and consistent pursuit of both these objectives, not merely one of them, that distinguishes group work as a process" (p. 291).

Newstetter further stressed the importance of maintaining this dual emphasis. He wrote, "Unless there is the combined and consistent pursuit of both objectives, the efforts do not fall entirely within this concept of group work. The underlying social-philosophical assumption is that individualized growth and social ends are interwoven and interdependent; that individuals and their social environment are equally important" (pp. 296-297).

Middelman (1982) and Wright (1999) have explored the potential that social work groups have when they incorporate programming. Programming assists group members to express themselves in non-verbal or alternative ways, thus encouraging a healthy progression toward the group's purpose. Additionally, it can assist in maintaining the balance between individual growth and social ends when used conscientiously with the stages of group development in mind.

A self-defense class is a social work group. It fosters a supportive peer relationship that can change women's lives. Many women who enroll in a self-defense class have been victimized in some way. Not only are they looking for a way to feel safe again, they are also looking for a way to re-connect socially. This pursuit of individual growth and social connection make a self-defense class worthwhile and, ultimately, a therapeutic experience.

A self-defense class can be a legitimate intervention to use for women who have been victimized. Yet, it is often not included in the menu of services offered to traumatized women. Therefore, the purpose of this article is to increase the awareness of the value a self-defense class can have when it incorporates basic group work principles. Seen in this light, a self-defense class gains an added weight and depth that can be appealing and helpful to women recovering from trauma.

Examples from the author's personal experiences and observations will be used to describe how a self-defense class is similar to a social work group. The type of self-defense class being discussed is an intensive five-week, 20-hour class, consisting of approximately 12-15 female participants. Verbal skills like boundary setting as well as non-verbal self-defense techniques are used in role-plays where women are put into an adrenalized state. The adrenalized state is a re-enactment of a dangerous and stressful situation a woman might face such as a robbery or a rape. In the adrenalized state, a woman's anxiety level is so high it often creates an inability to think or act decisively. This is also known as the freeze response where a woman is literally frozen and does not know what to do (Ellensweig, 1997). By repeatedly putting women into the adrenalized state, they become accustomed to the multitude of emotions that arise and learn how to think and act clearly to avoid getting hurt.

The class also includes the use of a female instructor and at least one male instructor who acts as the assailant in a padded suit. The majority of documented sexual violence against women is perpetrated by men. Having a male instructor act as the potential assailant adds a heightened sense of reality to the situation. Additionally, being padded allows women to apply the self-defense techniques they are learning to target areas of the assailant's body with full force and power.

Literature regarding self-defense and other groups used to address the needs of women suffering from trauma will be explored. Conceptual frameworks used in group work will also be discussed. It is important to note that this article is not stating that a self-defense class should be used in place of other forms of psychotherapy for women suffering from trauma. Nor is it implying that self-defense teachers should be viewed as social group workers, equipped with the specific skills and knowledge that social workers have. Self-defense teachers do take on many of the positive characteristics that social workers emulate. Kurland and Salmon (1993) have noted that teachers are excellent role models for social workers, specifically in terms of their passion for learning and their ability to be perceived as humanly fallible by their students (p. 166). These characteristics are utilized by self-defense teachers to help engage group members and can reflect tenets of social work practice. Therefore, this paper will focus on the unique group dynamic created by a self-defense class and how important that dynamic is to women completing the class successfully.

LITERATURE REVIEW

Group work has been cited frequently as an excellent intervention to be used by women suffering from PTSD and other trauma-related conditions. Many women who have experienced a trauma, such as a rape or sexual assault, feel and exhibit a variety of symptoms: re-experiencing of the trauma, frightening thoughts, hyper-vigilance or hyper-arousal, irritability, aggressiveness, withdrawal from people, places and things that were once pleasurable, isolation, guilt, low self-esteem and emotional numbness (Harvard University, 2005; National Center for PTSD, 2005; National Institute of Mental Health, 2005; PTSD Alliance, 2005; Foa, Keane, and Friedman, 2000; Watson, Scott and Regalsky, 1996).

One effective intervention recommended for PTSD is intensive psychotherapy, such as exposure therapy or Cognitive Behavior Therapy or C.B.T. (National Center of PTSD, 2005). In these approaches, the woman recalls the traumatic experience in a safe and contained environment where she can learn how to relax and cope with the memory itself. C.B.T. can improve a person's sense of self-control and personal safety by lessening the intense anxiety associated with the trauma (Harvard University, 2005; Foa, Keane, and Friedman, 2000).

Group interventions are also highly recommended to combat the isolation and stigma that comes with a trauma. When women meet other women who have experienced a similar trauma, they form a type of bond or "sisterhood" that can be extremely beneficial. As Foa, Keane, and Friedman (2000) describe, " . . . by encouraging group members repeatedly to experience their personal tragic events, as well as being exposed vicariously to the experiences of other group members, the model incorporates trauma processing" (p. 159). Women become witnesses for one another, validating the experience and the feelings associated with trauma.

A number of different types of groups have been used for this population. Carey (1998) analyzed a group for child abuse survivors and describes it as an opportunity for the group to affirm and humanize the victim, thus taking away the shame she may feel. He notes that when members share their story, they re-claim the power and control lost through the experience. Watson, Scott, and Regalsky (1996) focused on a group that includes two facilitators who made the group a safe space in which members could decrease the self-blame accompanying their trauma. Foa, Keane, and Friedman (2000) note that groups of all kinds, including drama or creative therapy groups, are especially helpful to individuals affected by trauma. The art of performing can help improve a woman's self-esteem and decrease her feelings of shame.

Self-defense training meets many of the needs and recommendations for women with trauma because it incorporates aspects of varying psychotherapy methods in a group setting. Ellensweig (1997) reported that the class may improve self-esteem and self-protection skills for women. A longitudinal study on self-defense graduates by Hollander (2004) revealed that women felt much more comfortable interacting with strangers and intimates because of their experience in a self-defense class.

Daniels (2001) studied a group of survivors of child sexual abuse who participated in a self-defense class in addition to a traditional psychotherapy group. The women reported improvements in their feelings of empowerment and decreased levels of anxiety and depression. Although this could be attributed to the use of group psychotherapy, Anderson (1999) has written that psychotherapy does not deal directly with the physical aspects of healing, as a self-defense class does. He goes on to state that adding physicality to treatment can provide, ". . . an emotional intensity to the experience [trauma] through eliciting anger and fear and providing an opportunity for memories to resurface." Ambrosia (2003) has also noted that a self-defense class is " . . . an excellent adjunct to psychotherapy." It parallels many of the same concepts discussed in therapy such as clear boundary setting, confronting challenging life situations and feeling empowered. Similarly, Brecklin and Ullman (2004) write that the therapeutic benefits to self-defense training include decreases in psychological distress, fear, vulnerability, anxiety, avoidance, and helplessness.

Because of the intense emotions elicited in a self-defense class, there are many variables which must be taken into account when planning and implementing a self-defense class. Ellensweig (1997) writes that the common response to an attack is a paralysis or ineffective flailing. Self-defense training would then need to incorporate re-enactments of threatening situations in an adrenalized state, allowing women to think and act in frightening scenarios. Brown (1995) has also discussed this common reaction, calling it the freeze response to an inappropriate situation. He notes that a self-defense class is more than just learning a few simple kicks and punches; it is deciding what you are willing to fight for. Brecklin and Ullman (2004) recommended that a self-defense class teach techniques that are practical, effective and simple. Madden and Sokol (1997) write that women's sizes and strengths must be taken into consideration. Rather than focusing on all upper body techniques, the class should include many lower body techniques, as women carry a lot of strength and power in their hips and thighs. It is crucial that padded, male instructors be present to practice these techniques. They go on to note that a self-defense class is not a martial arts class, though it can be commonly viewed as one. A self-defense class, unlike a martial arts class, takes into consideration the emotional ramifications of defending one's life.

The physical aspects combined with the therapeutic value of a self-defense class create a unique experience for women, grounded in group work concepts. Fraser and Russell (2000) conducted a study on the role of the group in relation to women's ability to grasp self-defense skills. The women interviewed consistently reported that the group was critical in their success with the class. The class encouraged positive interaction with victories becoming a collective rather than an individual experience. The group was there to "hold" the emotions of the woman fighting, similar to the way in which groups for trauma survivors act as witnesses. Additionally, women reported that watching fights over and over again desensitized them to the violence and, watching women win the fights over and over again, made them feel that they too would be able to win their own fights.

What the women in the study describe about a self-defense class is what is at the heart of social group work. Groups in which there is an activity have a two part purpose to them: doing the activity and then discussing what came out of the activity for individuals and the group as a whole (Kaplan, 2001; Northen and Kurland, 2001). The activity itself provides an opportunity to communicate emotions, explore problem solving techniques and improve self-esteem. As Wright (1999) notes, personal growth comes not just from mastering the skills but also from the cognitive recognition of the complexity of the experience of using the skill (p. 33). Groups also present members with the opportunity to explore other roles they may eventually take on in their daily lives. They aim to help members integrate what Shulman (1999) calls the outer self, presented in social situations, with the inner self, the true person within. Groups promote healthy roles that are for the good of the group and discourage unhealthy roles which can put the group at a disadvantage (Northen and Kurland, 2001). What ties all of these group work elements together is the use of mutual aid. Defined by Steinberg (2004) as people helping people as they think things through, mutual aid is at the heart of groups. Mutual aid creates an atmosphere where members can try new ways of thinking, being and doing. It is these group work principles that fuel a self-defense class and contribute to its paralleling of a social work group.

DISCUSSION

There are three ways that a self-defense class mirrors a social work group: its use of stages of group development, its ability to confront member roles, and its reliance on mutual aid.

Stages of Group Development

A self-defense class is essentially an activity-based social work group that uses specific programming to accomplish its dual purpose.

This dual purpose is to help members learn self-defense techniques *and* to help members feel safe and secure in their lives. As Northen and Kurland (2001) wrote, "Activity is not just busy work for a group, not used merely as a way to keep group members occupied. Rather, when thinking about activity, social workers need to assess the usefulness of a particular activity in furthering the group's purpose" (p. 282). The structure of the class, therefore, tunes into the stages of group development, acknowledging what members will need from a beginnings, middles and endings perspective to help accomplish its purpose.

Beginnings

In the beginning of any group, members feel nervous, anxious and uncertain. They are dependent on the facilitator to ease them into the group and create a safe environment. These are the same fears women face during their first self-defense class with much of their attention focused on the prospect of having to fight. Women are especially intimidated and lean on the self-defense instructors to explain how the class will unfold.

The first class starts with an opening circle where members take turns sharing why they have made the decision to take a self-defense course. This is where the instructors tune into the general vibe of the group and what the individual purposes are for each member. These individual purposes will be fused with the group's overall purpose as the class progresses. After each member has shared, the instructors then discuss the purpose of the class in great detail, offering the historical and conceptual frameworks that form the foundation of the group.

After this initial sharing, the rest of the first class consists of learning very basic self-defense techniques and then using them in slow, deliberate fights. The class is composed of three types of fights: front attacks, rear attacks and reversals. Front attacks are fights women can see coming at them. Rear attacks are surprise fights from behind. Reversals are rape scenarios where a woman may be pinned to the ground and will need to fight her way out. They are called reversals because the woman will eventually reverse the power the assailant feels he has.

Because of the unique nature and feelings that may emerge for each of these kinds of fights, the beginning stages of the group focus just on the front attacks. These are the most predictable and the least surprising. This is no accident; members are in the midst of the approach/avoidance stage and need to be taken care of by the instructors and not made to feel that they are clueless when it comes to defending themselves. Women learn clear and specific techniques and then apply them in a very controlled, slow, and deliberate way. During each fight, the female instructor is heavily involved, coaching the fighter as she demonstrates the techniques she has learned. Members are also encouraged to cheer on each woman during her fight. The members are leaning on the instructor to guide them through while they adjust to this new found way of thinking and being.

At the end of the first class, members re-group and discuss how the first night went for them. These opening and closing circles where women can share their feelings will happen during each class. This is when women do the talking part of an activity-based group. This is not a free-flow discussion and more often mirrors a "hot-seat" approach to sharing where a woman is put on the spot to say how she's feeling (Middleman and Wood, 1990). However, it still accomplishes the goal of women being able to express how their own personal purpose coincides with the group's overall purpose.

Erin exemplifies some of the common fears and concerns women face during the beginning of a self-defense class. In the following vignette from the opening circle of her class, she expresses her uncertainty:

> **Female Instructor:** *"Okay, why don't we take a moment to go around and have each of you introduce yourselves and tell us what brought you here tonight. Erin, since you're next to me, you get to go first."*

> **Erin:** *"All right. Hi everyone, my name is Erin. Um . . . I'm sorry, I am just so nervous (Laughs). I really didn't even want to come tonight. I mean, I signed up for this class because I felt I really needed it but I don't know if I can do this. Um . . . I was robbed outside of my apartment about three months ago and I thought I was totally fine afterwards. I didn't get hurt or anything. But, since then, I just . . . I don't know, I have been so paranoid and scared all the time. I mean, when I was robbed, it was like, I checked out. I didn't even know what was happening until it was over. So, I guess . . . I'm here to not be so scared anymore. And I have no idea how I'm going to . . . hit something. I'm a really quiet person and I'm not very physical so . . . I don't know, I guess we'll see what happens."*

By the end of the first class, Erin's fights seemed to alleviate some of her initial fears.

She again spoke openly during the closing circle:

Female Instructor: *"All right, Erin, you're next. How was tonight for you?"*

Erin: *"Wow. I feel awesome (Group laughs) I was so nervous when I came in here tonight and when you showed us that first fight we were going to do, I was like, no way! I mean, I had no idea how I was going to do all of that. It was really, really scary but after I did it, I was so happy. It felt so good to kick something (more laughter from group and Erin). Really, I feel great, just great. And I can't wait for next week."*

Female Instructor: *Excellent. "Great work tonight Erin."*

Middles

Group cohesiveness, establishment of trust, risk-taking and increased levels of intimacy are just a few of the many tasks members accomplish during the middle stages of a group. The comfort and security members feel at this particular moment of a group's life helps them to confront whatever challenges they face without fear of ridicule or rejection. These patterns of middle stages are no different in a self-defense class and are essentially mirrored through the way in which the fights change as well as how members interact with one another.

As the members grasp the overall concepts of self-defense, the fights begin to progress. Entering the beginning of the middles stage, front attacks are replaced with rear attacks which are more intense and frightening. The speed of the fighting begins to increase slightly. Verbal techniques are also incorporated into the class design as well. As women begin to find the hidden power in their bodies, they also find the hidden power in their voices. They learn the art of negotiation, practicing different verbal techniques that can ward off an attacker before he even reaches for her. At this point in the life of the group, women begin to trust each other and the instructors. As the fights increase in their degree of difficulty and danger, so too does the cohesiveness of the group itself. The connectedness between members intensifies as the fights intensify. Women become more involved in each other's fights and begin to cheer more during each fight.

Once in the heart of middles, fights have progressed to reversals. Reversals involve male instructors pinning women to the floor as if they are about to be raped. The male instructors also start talking to women during the fight, using provocative and manipulative language an assailant might use. The increase in the physical and verbal assault produces the greatest amount of emotion from women. They are at their most vulnerable during these scenarios. Therefore, it is imperative that the introduction of the reversal not take place until the group is in the middle stages. By then, members have reached a heightened level of intimacy and trust amongst each other. They feel safe enough to experience this frighteningly realistic scenario in front of the group, knowing they will receive support and encouragement.

As the journey through the latter part of middles continues, the fights become less predictable and more chaotic. Women are now relying more on themselves and each other and less on the instructors. Consequently, instructors pull back from being so specific and clear about what may happen in the next fight. Fights are soon improvised and women must integrate the verbal and non-verbal skills they have acquired. The sharing in the group's opening and closing circles also changes. Women speak more about how self-defense relates to other aspects of their lives. They speak more about how their personal purpose for taking the class is changing as the fights change. Fighting off a potential attacker in the class becomes an analogy for handling a difficult boss or needy friend. Successfully setting clear boundaries with a would-be assailant allows women to think of other boundaries they should set in their lives.

Continuing with the example of Erin, the following vignette from a middles closing circle illustrates the changes that have occurred in her and how she views the group:

Female Instructor: *"Erin, you're next. One thing that you loved about tonight and one thing you want to work on."*

Erin: *"Well . . ., um, this was really tough tonight. Those reversals were really scary and, not only when I was doing mine, but when I was seeing everyone else's fights. I mean, I got so emotional during everyone's fights, it was just so sad but, at the same time, it was so inspiring to see everyone get out of that. I . . . I feel so close to all of you having watched you do this. Anyway, one thing I loved about tonight, that I thought I did well in, was my reversal. There was a moment in it where I was like, 'Okay, this is it, I'm finished.' But I just kept fighting because everyone was cheering and I felt that suddenly there was hope. So, I'm proud of that. And, one thing I need to work on . . . those verbal scenarios. Those are sometimes even harder than the fights! I find that I really have trouble setting boundaries*

*with people and often, especially at my job, I end up doing things I
don't want to do. I'm staying late or I'm coming in on holidays. That
one scenario we did, that was so my boss (some laughter). So, yeah,
I need to work on that here and, really, in my life."*

Endings

The ending or termination stage of a group can be difficult. Members
regress slightly, returning to the initial fear and uncertainty they walked
into the group with (Garland, Jones, and Kolodny, 1973). Once again
they rely more on the facilitator to help them transition out of the group.
In a self-defense class members have grown attached to one another in a
very short amount of time. They have witnessed each other come out of
dangerous and traumatic situations victoriously. As a result, they feel
intimately linked and connected and are often wondering how they will
feel secure outside of the group. Members also worry if the self-defense
skills they have acquired will stay with them once the group is over.

The way the class can honor the multitude of feelings that endings
provokes is by holding a graduation. Graduation is a celebration of the
members' accomplishments. They invite friends and family to come
and watch them fight. Instructors give members two fights that they will
execute in front of their loved ones. These fights return to the fairly slow
and deliberate pace they started at. As with endings stages, instructors
also return to their beginning role of the nurturing and caring figure that
members can lean on. Instructors ensure that members look good in
front of an audience, thus showing members that they have been successful and can carry these skills with them when they leave the group.
After the graduation, the guests are asked to leave so the group can hold
their final closing circle. This closure is essential to allowing participants the opportunity to validate what they have learned and to thank
one another and the instructors for the opportunity.

Erin's emotional goodbye during the final closing circle again illustrates the journey she has taken from the beginning, through the middle,
to the end of the group:

Female Instructor: *"Erin, how was tonight for you?"*

Erin: *"I just feel so amazing. I, um, (begins to tear up) Wow, I really didn't think I was going to get emotional. I am just so proud of
us all tonight. We were so awesome! I feel so much safer and more
confident than I did when I walked in here. Not just in terms of*

physical safety but emotionally I feel like I know how to protect myself from being taken advantage of or feeling dismissed. This has helped me in so many ways and I feel so grateful to all of you. So, I made everyone little ribbons that say 'Number One Ass-Kicker.'" (Group laughs and applauds as Erin gives each member and instructors a ribbon.)

A self-defense class truly adheres to the stages of group development. Progressing from slow, deliberate and predictable fights to intense, aggressive and unpredictable fights, members see their own gradual improvement and the improvement of others. Without this specific structure for how fighting and group cohesiveness will unfold, members would have trouble believing in themselves as capable fighters.

Member Roles

There are four unique fighting roles that emerge in a self-defense class, similar to the traditional roles that emerge in other groups such as the scapegoat or the isolate. Each fighting role represents a different aspect of the self and how it can impede a woman's ability to defend herself in both a verbal and non-verbal way. The way a woman deals with everyday conflict is reflected in the way she handles dangerous and unpredictable conflict. During all fights, the female instructor continuously coaches the fighter. This is done while the women are also cheering on the fighter. The clear message to the members is that, regardless of what type of fighting role a woman may take on at any one moment, she is still a fighter. She has made the decision to fight for her life and she can win. Depending on what type of fight (front, rear, or reversal), women may take on any one of these roles throughout the life of the group.

The first role that may emerge is the *nay-saying fighter*, the member who does not believe the self-defense techniques will work. A nay-saying fighter generally has a defeatist attitude, looking at life through a pessimist's lens. An example of when the nay-saying fighter emerges is during rape scenarios where women are asked to throw off an assailant who has pinned them to the ground. Judy, a nay-saying fighter, had strong doubts when she first saw the reversal. During practice sessions, prior to her actual fight, she had trouble with the techniques and expressed her skepticism.

Male Instructor: *"Okay Judy, let's give this a try. I'm going to pin you and I want you to throw me off."*

Judy: *"All right, we'll see" (Judy is pinned and makes a half-hearted attempt to throw her assailant off, which proves unsuccessful).*

Male Instructor: *"Let's try it again."*

Judy: *"You're too heavy. I'm too small. This is impossible."*

Male Instructor: *"It's totally possible, you have a lot of strength and I know you can do this. I want you to yell no when you throw me off."*

Judy: *"No" (moves instructor off her slightly) "Oh, this isn't going to work. What if he's pinning me down and pulling my hair. What then?"*

Male Instructor: *"I promise you, you can throw me off, even if I'm doing all those things. I want you to try it again and really yell no. In fact, yell no right now."*

Judy: *"No!"*

Male Instructor: *"Again!"*

Judy: *"NO!"*

Male Instructor: *"Throw me off!"*

Judy: *"NO!" (Throws male instructor off) "Whoa." (laughs) "Okay, I guess that worked."*

Judy eventually went on to win her actual fight after getting over her belief that the technique was impossible. Nay-saying fighters typically ask instructors how to get out of very specific or detailed situations. It is important that the instructors continually focus on the fights happening in the moment. As the nay-saying fighter sees that the small techniques used in the class have big rewards, she soon understands that they will prevent worse situations from occurring.

The second role to develop is that of the *quiet fighter*. She does not yell loud and, therefore, does not hit hard. She has faith that others will be able to use the skills successfully, but that she will not. Whereas the nay-saying fighter lacks confidence in the self-defense skills, the quiet fighter lacks confidence in her self and does not try hard enough. Her self-doubt plays itself out in a fight and it is the members and instructors jobs to help the quiet fighter find her power. Susan is a typical quiet fighter who has particular difficulty speaking and yelling loudly during confrontation. She expressed early in the class that she has trouble sticking up for herself and often apologizes when she does. Her fighting style reflects this aspect of her personality. In the following scenario the group and instructors try to break her of her habit.

>   **Susan:** *(quietly) "No. Leave me alone."*

>   **Instructor:** *"Susan, I want you to say that again, louder."*

>   **Susan:** *"No! Leave me alone."*

>   **Instructor:** *"I don't believe you Susan, you need to be really loud, no need to apologize or be nice here."*

>   **Susan:** *"NO! LEAVE ME ALONE!"*

>   **Group:** *"That's right Susan, c'mon!"*

>   **Assailant:** *"No?" (mocking tone) 'No!' "Gimme a break!"*

>   **Susan:** *"No! Go away!"*

>   **Instructor:** *"Step in and knee!"*

>   **Susan and Group:** *"NO!"*

>   **Instructor:** *"Harder!"*

>   **Group:** *"Harder Susan, hit 'em hard!"*

>   **Susan:** *(As she hits) "NO! NO! NO!"*

>   **Instructor:** *(whistle blows) "He's out!"*

Group: *"Woo hoo! Awesome fight!"*

Susan saw that the instructor and her peers believed in her. The goading by the assailant also pushed her to find the inner strength she needed to overcome her struggle with being more assertive. Quiet fighters need to be prodded during fights. As a result, they give themselves permission to be a louder and more of a presence.

The third role is that of the *smiling fighter.* This fighter masks her fear in her smile; in nearly every fight she is smiling, even giggling to hide her nervousness. A smiling fighter admits to avoiding conflict as much as possible or making a joke out of it. She does not take the fights seriously and often laughs at what the assailants say to her, even during particularly difficult fights, such as rape scenarios. In Jennifer's case, the assailant used her smile against her, taking it to mean that she was not serious about wanting him to leave her alone.

Assailant: *"I like that smile. I could take you home, make you smile all night."*

Jennifer: *(smiles) "No"*

Assailant: *"Aw, you don't mean that sweetheart."*

Instructor: *"Jennifer, this is not a joke."*

Jennifer: *"I know it's not, I can't help it."*

Instructor: *"Yes you can."*

Group: *"C'mon Jennifer, you can do it."*

Jennifer: *(rolls her eyes, giggles) "Ugh! I don't know what to do."*

Instructor: *"Take a breath. This guy is serious. I want you to look at him and listen to what he's saying to you."*

Assailant: *"You want to go home with me? Huh? C'mon beautiful, let's get in my car and go."*

> **Jennifer:** *(takes a deep breath)* *"No. Turn around and walk away."*

> **Instructor:** *"Good."*

> **Group:** *"Nice, nice, yeah."*

When Jennifer saw that everyone else in the room was taking the fight seriously, she decided to do the same. The assailant would not let her make a joke out of their interaction. This focus helped her engage in the scenario and commit to winning the fight. Smiling fighters need to face and handle the conflicts presented to them and not be allowed to find the easy way out.

The fourth role is the *scared fighter* who often cries or freezes up during a fight. She often has been through a traumatic experience already and fights may bring up some deep-seated feelings of re-living the trauma itself. She often feels or perhaps even is the perpetual victim. The scared fighter, similar to the quiet fighter, also lacks confidence in herself, but the origin of such lack of confidence may stem from a particularly traumatic episode in her past. The following vignette with Pam, who is a survivor of a sexual assault, illustrates how upset the scared fighter becomes in the moment:

> **Assailant:** *"Hey baby! Tonight is your lucky night–I'm taking you home!"*

> **Pam:** *"No!" (Begins to cry) "I can't do this."*

> **Instructor:** *"Yes you can, Pam."*

> **Group:** *"We're with you Pam, you're not alone, you can do this."*

> **Instructor:** *"You're gonna step in and knee him. It's okay to cry. You can fight and cry at the same time, nobody ever said you couldn't."*

> **Group:** *"Get 'em Pam"*

> **Pam:** *"No! Go away."*

> **Instructor:** *"That's it, keep going."*

The instructor and the group reassure Pam that she does not have to be the victim for the rest of her life. Scared fighters must go through the fights, regardless of how similar they may be to an event in their own lives. By re-experiencing the trauma in a different way where she comes out the winner, the scared fighter will see that her trauma does not have to define her.

Mutual Aid

Mutual aid is at the heart of a self-defense class and connects women to one another in a unique way. Women share their thoughts and feelings during the opening and closing circle of the group. This can be helpful in that it gives them the opportunity to check in with themselves, hear from other members and know that their experience in the class is a shared one. However, women help each other *during* the fights more than any other time of a self-defense class. From the very first slow and steady fight, women are encouraged to "be with the fighter," supporting her throughout her fight, from start to finish. There are four ways that mutual aid is encouraged during fights.

First, before every fight, women huddle up and dedicate the fight to some concept or idea. The dedication is for something they will aspire to do, like hitting hard, or reject, like freezing up during a fight. This is a way for the women to come together as a whole and know that when they go out for their fight, they will not be alone. It helps to calm the jitters many women experience before each fight. Most important, it involves applying individual purposes to the group's overall purpose. One woman's own struggle or goal in a fight becomes everyone's struggle.

Instructor: *"So, does anyone have a dedication for this fight?"*

Marlene: *"To staying calm?"* *(Group nods approvingly).*

Instructor: *"Okay Marlene, I like that, to staying calm. Count it off for us."*

Marlene: *"Three, two, one!"*

Group: *"Yes! Yes! Yes!"*

With their arms wrapped around each other in a traditional sports huddle, women give each other squeezes and nods of encouragement and support. They get excited for their own fights and for each other's.

The second way women help each other during each fight is that they are asked to keep their "toes to the mat" which literally means to put your toes to the edge of the mat, rather than sit back against the wall watching the fight from a distance while waiting for your turn. By stepping up to the edge of the mat and engaging in what is happening in front of them, they also become a part of that fight. They bear witness to the process the woman fighting is going through. Not only is this helpful to the woman fighting but also to the women waiting for their turn to fight. Watching a fight unfold can be a powerful experience for members. As Naomi said during the class, "When I'm watching other women fighting, I feel like I'm a part of their fight. I feel uncomfortable, scared and angry with them. I want to jump in there and fight with her."

"Toes to the mat" segues into the third way mutual aid is achieved during fights: cheering. Perhaps the single most important thing that women do for one another during each and every fight is to cheer. The cheering and yelling of the women on the mat helps to fuel the fighter, reminding her that she too has the capacity to yell no against her attacker and knock him out.

Instructor: "*Step in and knee.*"

Fighter and Group: "*NO!*"

Instructor: "*Step in and eyes.*"

Fighter and Group: "*NO!*"

Group member 1: "*All right Catherine!*"

Group member 2: "*C'mon Catherine!*"

Fighter: "*NO!*"

Again, this is a reciprocal relationship. Women who are in the midst of their fight feel the connection with the women watching them as they yell with every move they perform. Women watching the fight and cheering the fighter on also get something out of the fight. "I love the cheering almost as much as the fighting," said Elizabeth, "It helps me to connect with the woman fighting and it gets out a lot of my own aggression and anxiety before my own fight."

Finally, the fourth way women help each other during fights is by winning them. Women must fight their fights until the attacker is knocked out. This means that, as the class progresses and women become savvier in the art of self-defense, they are given more challenging fights, which may take longer to win. But, the fights are always won. As a result, women not fighting are continuously exposed to seeing other women fight off attackers and rapists. Seeing this over and over again eventually instills in them that they too will be able to win their fight, even if it looks close to impossible. Women see reflections of themselves on the mat when they are not fighting. They see themselves victorious time and time again. It becomes an intensely emotional and empowering moment when each woman wins her fight. As Carla noted in one closing circle, "When one of you wins a fight, I get a lump in my throat. I am so moved that it's like I've won the fight, too."

RECOMMENDATIONS AND CONCLUSION

When a self-defense class acknowledges how social group work principles affect group process and use this knowledge in planning, it gains added weight and legitimacy. A self-defense class is not only an opportunity to learn a practical, physical skill: it is an opportunity for connection and healing. Self-defense classes could be utilized much more by the helping profession. The therapeutic benefits of this class are unique and deserve further exploration, particularly by those in the field of trauma therapy. Self-defense classes could be a wonderful, short-term intervention, allowing survivors to jump large hurdles in a small period of time.

Not all self-defense classes incorporate group work principles. Therefore, before referring clients to a self-defense class, preliminary screening should take place to determine if it is a good fit. Kurland (1982) addressed the art of screening and wrote, "In talking with people and in surveying past and present services, themes will begin to emerge. Such themes and comments are often the starting points for the development of groups" (p. 12). Questions one might ask about a potential self-defense group could include the following: Is there a male and female instructor? Are verbal and non-verbal skills utilized? Do the members participate in role-plays while in an adrenalized state? What type of helping relationship is established between the members? How does this relationship change over the course of the class? How does the group address the individual challenges each member faces? How does the first class differ from the last class?

A self-defense class can be a powerful group experience. When it incorporates basic group work principles such as stages of group development, member roles and mutual aid, it becomes an amazing and transformational experience for its members. Adding a self-defense class to the repertoire of services available to women who have experienced trauma will provide a valuable and beneficial opportunity to help them heal and recover.

REFERENCES

Ambrosia, P. (2003). *Model mugging: How does a women's self-defense course inform psychotherapy?* (Doctoral dissertation. Antioch U/New England Graduate School, 2003). Dissertations Abstracts International, 63, 10-B.

Anderson, K. (1999). *Healing the fighting spirit: Combining self-defense training and group therapy for women who have experienced incest.* (Doctoral dissertation. University of Minnesota, 1999). Dissertation Abstracts International, 59, 9-B.

Brecklin, L. and Ullman, S. (2004). Correlates of post-assault self-defense/assertiveness training participation for sexual assault survivors. *Psychology of Women Quarterly*, 28, 147-158.

Brown, H. (1995). The myths and realities of self-defense training. *Total Health*, 17 (2), 44-47.

Carey, L. (1998). Illuminating the process of a rape survivors' support group. *Social Work with Groups*, 21(1/2), 103-116.

Daniels, K. (2001). *A program incorporating self-defense training and group therapy in the treatment of adult child sexual abuse survivors.* (Doctoral dissertation. University of Hartford, 2001). Dissertation Abstracts International, 62, 1-B.

Ellensweig, D. (1997). Never again: Model mugging: A therapeutic resource for the psychiatric nurse. *Journal of Psychosocial Nursing and Mental Health Services*, 35 (6), 41-47.

Foa, E., Keane, T., and Friedman, M. (2000). *Effective treatments for PTSD*. New York: Guilford Press.

Fraser, K. and Russell, G. (2000). The role of the group in acquiring self-defense skills: Results of a qualitative study. *Small Group Research*, 31 (4), 397-423.

Garland, J., Jones, H., and Kolodny, R. (1973). A model for stages of group development in social work groups. *Explorations in group work*, Bernstein (Ed.), Boston: Milford House, 17-71.

Harvard University. (2005). Not getting over it: Post-traumatic stress disorder. *Harvard Women's Health Watch*, March.

Hollander, J. (2004). I can take care of myself. *Violence Against Women*, 10(3), 205-216.

Kaplan, C. (2001). The purposeful use of performance in groups: A new look at the balance of task and process. *Social Work with Groups*, 24 (2), 47-67.

Kurland, R. (1982). Group formation: A guide to development of successful groups. Kinney, T. and Loavenbruck, G. (Eds.), *United Neighborhood Centers of America, Inc. and Continuing Education Program School of Social Welfare, Nelson A. Rockefeller College of Public Affairs and Policy, State University of New York at Albany*, 1-20.

Kurland, R. and Salmon, R. (1993). Not just one of the gang: Group workers and their role as an authority. Ephross, R. and Vassil, T. (Eds.), *Social Work with Groups: Expanding Horizons*, The Haworth Press, Inc., 153-169.

Madden, M. and Sokol, T. (1997). Teaching women self-defense: Pedagogical issues. *Feminist Teacher*, 11 (2), 133-152.

Middleman, Ruth. (1980). The use of program: Review and update. *Social Work with Groups*, 3 (3), 5-23.

Middleman, R. and Wood, G. G. (1990). *Skills for direct practice in social work*. New York: Columbia University Press.

National Center for PTSD. (2005). Treatment of PTSD, Retrieved February 21, 2005, from http://www.ncptsd.org/facts/treatments/fs_treatment.html

National Institute of Mental Health. (2005). *Post-Traumatic Stress Disorder*, Retrieved April 7, 2005, from http://www.nimh.gov/HealthINformation/ptsdmenu.cfm

Newstetter, W.I. (1935). What is social group work? *Proceedings of the National Conference of Social Work*, 291-299.

Northen, H. and Kurland, R. (2001). *Social work with groups* (3rd ed.). New York: Columbia University Press.

PTSD Alliance. (2005). *What are the symptoms of PTSD?*, Retrieved April 7, 2005, from http://www.ptsdalliance.org/about_symp.html

Shulman, L. (1999). *The skills of helping individuals, families, groups, and communities* (4th ed.). Itasca: F.E. Peacock Publishers, Inc

Steinberg, D. (2004). *The mutual-aid approach to working with groups* (2nd ed.). New York: The Haworth Press, Inc.

Watson, G., Scott, C., and Ragalsky, S. (1996). Refusing to be marginalized: Group work in mental health services for women survivors of childhood sexual abuse. *Journal of Community & Applied Social Psychology*, 6, 341-354.

Wright, W. (1999). The use of purpose in on-going activity groups: A framework for maximizing the therapeutic impact. *Social Work with Groups*, 15 (4), 3-14.

I'm Gone When You're Gone: How a Group Can Survive When Its Leader Takes a Leave of Absence

Joanna Pudil

SUMMARY. As the roles and demands on social workers increase in their agencies and their personal lives, there is a greater chance that they will need to take a leave of absence. This is also true for social workers who lead groups. This article presents a process to allow the primary worker to take a leave of absence while the group continues with an interim worker. The author's personal experience of a leave of absence from a HIV+ adolescent support group will be used to illustrate this transfer process. In providing ample time and a thoughtful process of transfer, this leave of absence was successful in maintaining group attendance and participation. *[Article copies available for a fee from The Haworth Document Delivery Service: 1-800-HAWORTH. E-mail address: <docdelivery@haworthpress.com> Website: <http://www.HaworthPress.com> © 2006 by The Haworth Press, Inc. All rights reserved.]*

KEYWORDS. Stage of development, HIV/AIDS, adolescents, termination, transfer, support groups

---

[Haworth co-indexing entry note]: "I'm Gone When You're Gone: How a Group Can Survive When Its Leader Takes a Leave of Absence." Pudil, Joanna. Co-published simultaneously in *Social Work with Groups* (The Haworth Press, Inc.) Vol. 29, No. 2/3, 2006, pp. 217-233; and: *Making Joyful Noise: The Art, Science, and Soul of Group Work* (ed: Andrew Malekoff, Robert Salmon, and Dominique Moyse Steinberg) The Haworth Press, Inc., 2006, pp. 217-233. Single or multiple copies of this article are available for a fee from The Haworth Document Delivery Service [1-800-HAWORTH, 9:00 a.m. - 5:00 p.m. (EST). E-mail address: docdelivery@haworthpress.com].

doi:10.1300/J009v29n02_14

When a group member leaves an established ongoing group by choice or necessity, the remaining members must deal with the emotions associated with the loss of this member. The worker's role in these circumstances is to help the remaining members process and come to terms with the loss. There is a sense of finality to this departure, just as there is when life circumstances cause the worker to leave permanently. This happens with regularity when the group facilitator is a graduate social work student. At the end of the academic year, the student intern leaves. Considerable group work literature on termination exists. That includes the worker's role in this stage of group development (see, for example, Kurland and Salmon, 1998; Brandler and Roman, 1999; and Northern and Kurland, 2001).

However, there are also times when the group worker must take an extended leave of absence from the agency and is replaced temporarily by another staff member, until the original staff member returns and resumes her previous position and role. The issues of loss or separation, replacement, renewal and changes in roles are more complex in these circumstances. This paper presents an extended case example of the impact on group life when a worker takes a leave of absence and then returns.

EXPOSITION

As personal and professional demands increase in the lives of social workers, the reasons a group worker may need to take a leave of absence from the agency and the groups she leads also increase. These reasons may include maternity leave, educational training, medical leave or any opportunity that takes the worker away from the group for a substantial period of time. This paper will describe five steps that should be planned and implemented when a leave of absence is known in advance. These are as follows:

1. Providing ample time for the announcement of the primary worker's (hereinafter referred to as "PW") leaving.
2. Developing a system of transfer through meetings between the interim worker (hereinafter referred to as "IW") and primary workers.
3. Introducing the group members to the IW.
4. Processing group member's feelings and reactions about the transfer.

5. Reintroducing the group members to the PW when the leave of absence ends and the IW departs.

This paper is based on the author's own experience of taking a leave of absence due to maternity leave. The group, used to illustrate the five steps listed above, is an adolescent and young adult HIV+ support group led by this author. The support group is made up of male and female patients aged 18-26. The group is held at a clinic where the group members receive outpatient medical treatment. The members are able to meet with their medical provider and eat lunch before each group meeting. There are seven core members of the group. The group is open to anyone who comes to the clinic for services. The members are primarily African American and Hispanic young adults who live in poor, urban neighborhoods. The majority of the group members contracted HIV through sexual contact rather than at birth. The group had been meeting weekly for one year before the PW took a leave of absence.

LITERATURE REVIEW

There has been a considerable amount of social work literature written about termination within a group (Siebold, 1991; McGee, 1974; Malekoff, 1997; Northen and Kurland, 2001; Brandler and Roman, 1999; and Maholick and Turner, 1979). However, articles that focus on a group worker taking an extended leave of absence, then returning are conspicuously absent. A majority of the termination articles focus on the exit of the patients or clients. Northen and Kurland (2001) state that the social worker can also be the person who terminates the relationship. There are points of time in a therapeutic relationship when the worker may have to leave before the clients/patients have completed their treatment. McGee (1974) also states that the worker's termination from the group has rarely been examined in literature. McGee (1974) illustrates situations that may cause a worker to have to terminate with their group. Many of these situations (e.g., pregnancy and childbirth, illness, or leave of absence) do not necessarily mean that permanent termination is inevitable. Some workers were able to resume their work upon returning from the leave of absence. Malekoff (2004) states that the role of the worker in the termination phase is to provide a good transition from the group to a new worker. It must be "well timed, thoughtfully conceived and sensitively facilitated" (p. 188). This is also true in the transfer process to an IW when the PW takes a leave of absence.

It has been stated that termination within a group "is the microcosmic representation of some of life's most crucial and painful issues" (Yalom, 1995, p. 373). Thus, it has been duly noted in the literature that the termination process within a group needs to be conducted with much care and consideration for the group. Vichnis (1999) states that members' "responses to terminations can be based on residual feelings from past transitional experiences, such as the divorce of one's parents, children growing up and leaving home, or the death of a loved one" (p. 144). Common feelings that can arise include fear, anger, rejection, guilt, loss, and frustration (McGee, 1974; Mackenzie, 1996). It has been the author's experience that these reactions and feelings may occur when the group leader takes a leave of absence.

Vichnis (1999) further examines the process of transition and the impact on a group when a worker takes a leave of absence. This change can be difficult for members because of the uncertainty of their relationship with the new worker. It is as if they are suspended and left dangling emotionally until the PW returns. A well planned transfer, however, allows the group to be firmly grounded before the known worker leaves, increasing the possible continued success of the group.

ANNOUNCING THE LEAVE

A PW needs to give the group as much notice as possible in order to give the members time to come to terms emotionally with her temporary departure. Providing little or no notice is destructive to the group (McGee, 1974). As Siebold (1991) states, "one way to help patients accept reality is to give them sufficient facts so that they can master the news, and then allow them as much time to process this information" (p. 194). Therefore, the PW needs to inform the group of her leaving as soon as possible. She should also relay the terms of the leave such as length, dates, and who the IW will be. Informing the group may occur even before the complete transfer process is settled, such as the identity of the new worker when that is known. As Vichnis (1999) states, it is "important to maintain an open and honest dialogue with the group during the transferring process" (p. 146). This will provide ample time to assess the group members' initial reactions to the announcement:

> *PW*: I have an announcement for the group. (Members direct attention to the worker) I'm pregnant.

Nancy: That's great!

Christina: Wow, when are you due?

PW: I'm due the first week of October.

Akira: Does that make you five months pregnant?

John: Do you know what you're having?

Nancy: (looking at the group members) Let her talk.

PW: Yes, I'm five months pregnant and no, I don't know the sex of the baby.

Zaria: Shouldn't you know by now?

PW: Yes, I could if I wanted to, but I would be happy with a boy or a girl.

Zaria: But how are you going to know what clothes to buy?

Akria: You just buy lots of green, yellow and red clothing. Colors that a boy and girl can wear.

Nancy: I don't like those colors, that's why I chose to find out the sex when I was pregnant.

Akira and Zaria: (shake their heads in agreement)

Kim: So, how long are you going to be gone for? How long is maternity leave?

Christina: You're coming back right?

PW: Maternity leave is three months. It will begin the day I deliver, which is most likely my due date, October 3, so I will be back the second week of January.

Akira: What does this mean for the group? Who will be the program social worker?

PW: Well, I would hope the group continues on during my leave.

Zaria: How is that going to happen?

PW: The program is in the process of hiring a second social worker who will cover the group and all the cases at the program while I am on leave.

Akira: I hate getting to know new people. I will just work with Dr. C until you return.

Christina: I agree. I'm gone when you're gone (most group members nod their heads in agreement).

In this case the group members initially expressed resistance and resentment about the announcement of the leave of absence. In fact, the members' reactions had made the PW feel as if she had betrayed them. She was overwhelmed by this feeling and amazed at how quickly the members were willing to break up the group once the impending absence began. She feared that all her hard work to establish this group would easily end when she left and was expecting resistance. Instead, she was met with statements of complete abandonment from the group. The goal in discussing the leave of absence with them was to help keep the group together so that they would be able to continue to meet, because she feared that if the group stopped meeting it would be difficult to bring them back together again. In fact, it had been difficult to get the group started in the first place, and if they stopped meeting it would be as if they were throwing away all the hard work and accomplishments that they had achieved during the last year.

The PW soon realized that this was a unique opportunity to show members that someone can go away and come back, that a leave of absence did not mean their whole relationship had to be terminated. Thus, she turned her attention to the need to keep the group functioning during the leave of absence. By giving four months' notice of the impending leave of absence, she allowed the group members the time to work through the inherent difficulties of the transfer process. Because no one knew who the IW would be at the time, the choice to either tell the group with ample notice or to wait for the agency to hire a new social worker was difficult to make. Ultimately, the PW decided that waiting for the new social worker to be hired before announcing the leave would leave too little time to process with the group members. It would cause great anxiety among the group members, but this anxiety would dissipate if they used the extra time to work out the feelings and solidify a transfer plan while waiting for the new worker to be hired. The PW's decision to inform the group at this early point is supported by McGee (1974) who states, "when a worker plans to terminate, the operation and maintenance of the group should be given high priority" (p. 7).

DEVELOPING A SYSTEM OF TRANSFER

As Northen and Kurland (2001) state, "When a worker leaves before the group is ready to terminate, the desirable situation is a planned transfer to another worker. The amount of time it takes to accomplish a successful transfer depends on the nature of the group" (p. 303). Further, Vichnis (1999) states that when transferring the group from one worker to another, the IW and PW should meet to develop a plan of action. In fact, more than one meeting is essential in this process, because meetings provide the opportunity to share information, ask questions, and plan the actual transfer. In other words, transfer should be a collaborative effort if at all possible.

No group can remain the same when there is a transfer of workers, and it is important to establish planning meetings to develop a system of transfer. In the initial meeting, therefore, it is important to acquaint the IW with basic information, which can consist of group history, members and their roles, meeting time and day, and finally, group culture and norms. Also, the workers should decide on the number of planning meetings to have in order to facilitate the transfer process. In this case, a joint decision was made in the initial meeting to meet weekly until the leave of absence began.

It is also important for the workers to discuss their roles in the transfer, the timing of it, potential changes to the group, and how to incorporate the IW. During the meetings, there should be opportunities to communicate and give feedback on the progress of the transfer, which gives the IW a firm foundation for taking over and ensuring greater transitional success. In this case, the PW was concerned about the group members' resistance toward the IW and the group's continuing during her absence, and she had time to express those concerns during the planning meetings and to discuss the issues with the IW, who had the same concerns.

Over the course of these meetings the decision was made to change the group from a support group to an activity group. Since the IW was new to the program, it was anticipated that group members would not feel comfortable talking in depth about their personal lives. An activity group, however, would allow members to continue to meet but to focus on an activity rather than feel pressured to expose themselves to a new worker. Therefore, a list was developed of possible activities based on the IW's strengths and skills, and as a result, the two workers were able to make a clear and unified presentation to the group.

INTRODUCING THE GROUP TO THE INTERIM WORKER

The first meeting between the group and the IW should be brief. This allows them to meet her and then discuss their reactions after she leaves (Vichnis, 1999). As in the following excerpt, the contact with the IW can begin with a simple introduction.

PW: I would like to begin group today by introducing Doris, who is the new social worker at Project STAY.

Group members: (in a low mumble) Hello.

PW: Doris would you like to take a moment to introduce yourself?

IW: Hi. As Joanna said, I'm Doris. I just started at Project STAY this week. Even though I'm new to Project STAY, I've been in the hospital system for 10 years working in the school based clinics. At that job I worked with high school students individually and in group settings. I'm excited to be here.

PW: I would like to go around the room and have each member introduce themselves. Who would like to begin?

Nancy: I will. My name is Nancy. I have a daughter. I've been in the group since it began.

Christina: My name is Christina. I have no children. I live in Brooklyn with my mother. I just joined the group.

Akira: I'm Akira. I have one daughter and I'm currently pregnant. I live in Manhattan. I've been in the program for a long time and I don't like new people.

John: Hey, I'm John. I just came back from California.

Manny: I'm Manny. Welcome to the program. I've been in Project STAY for a long time.

Zaria: I'm Zaria. I have a daughter. I don't know what else to say.

Kim: Hi, I'm Kim. I've been with Dr. C for a long time. I live in Manhattan.

Lisa: (softly) I'm Lisa.

PW: Now that everyone has introduced themselves, does anyone have any questions for Doris? (Group members all shake their heads no.) Okay, Doris is going to leave and she will be coming back in a few weeks to begin discussing with the group what you would like to do during this time when she takes over the group. We will be co-leading the group for the last four weeks before I leave for maternity leave.

IW: Thank you for taking the time to meet me. I look forward to getting to know you all.

By keeping the first meeting brief, these group members were able to have time during the meeting to express their initial responses. They were civil but also guarded in what they said. Once the IW left, however, the members began voicing their initial impressions. They stated their dislike for her and her laid back, quiet personality. The members decided that she was too different and would not be able to meet their needs, alarming the PW, but it is important to remember they were still reacting to the idea that the PW was taking a leave of absence. Also, because a large number of members kept their HIV status a secret, they had historically tried to keep new people at a distance, automatically assuming that new people would be judgmental and reject them; in fact, they had been in situations that regularly exposed them to rejection. In order to preserve their sense of self, therefore, they tended to reject others before being rejected. The group members also felt this toward the IW, and the PW had to keep reminding herself that there was still time to work out these issues–that the transition could be successful and useful.

When a transfer is to be introduced, group members need ample time to get to know the new worker. Here, this was accomplished by co-leading a series of group meetings, allowing the members time to work out how the group would develop and change with a new worker. In the co-leading process, therefore, the IW also began to take the lead as the PW's date of departure loomed closer. It is also important for the two workers to meet after each co-led meeting to allow them to provide feedback and assist each other in fine tuning the transfer process.

Inviting group members to participate in the transfer process can assist them in getting to know an interim worker and is crucial to the introduction phase. It provides another way of developing the direction of the group and transfer by allowing members to have a voice. It also provides them with a greater sense of control over the transfer process. As Siebold (1991) sees it, there are three actors in the process of transfer: the therapist, the patient(s) and the future therapist. The workers may develop a planned direction for the group, but group members must have time to provide input into the new working agreement as well (Northen and Kurland, 2001), contributing to direction, purpose, and process. The opportunity to participate in the transfer process allows them to feel included in the change and invested in the outcome.

IW: I was wondering what the group would like to do during Joanna's maternity leave.

Nancy: What do you mean?

IW: I was thinking that we could change the group into an activity group while Joanna is out, since I'm new here and I'm still getting to know all of you.

Christina: Sounds good. What type of activity?

Kim: Let's watch movies.

Nancy: Yeah, I like that.

IW: We could do that or I know how to knit. I could teach you all how to knit.

Lisa: I already know how to knit.

Kim: I like that idea I could make Christmas presents for everyone.

Akira: Yeah, that's a good idea.

Providing these group members with a voice in the direction of the group during the leave of absence gave them a chance to open up and get to know the IW. The PW was concerned that they would keep their guard up and not be open to suggestions. However, after determining that the group would go from a therapeutic support group to a knitting activity group, the members appeared relieved and even excited about the new direction. They were open to and excited about learning to knit, permitting the IW to teach them a new skill. The easier choice for them would have been to watch movies, perhaps, during which there would be little interaction amongst themselves or with the IW. Instead, they chose to interact with her, and it began to appear as if a successful transition was possible.

PROCESSING FEELINGS AND REACTIONS

The responses that a group member may have toward a PW's leave and transfer process may range broadly (Vichnis, 1999). As Brandler and Roman (1991) say, the transfer/termination process may be a golden opportunity: how members act out their feelings around the termination reflects, for the worker, the member's previous separations. It provides a golden opportunity for the worker to consciously consider the past and the present by asking how this termination is like other losses in the member's life, how it is different, and what it recalls. This time a chance exists for the leave taking to be different from past separations and a chance to move the individual from the past into the present so that she may exercise control over her own (p. 84).

Vichnis (1999) adds that "this process allows the group members time to assess what achievements there have been, how purpose and goals changed as the group developed, and what work is still left unfinished" (p. 151). Much of this can be conducted through group members' reminiscence about group experiences, a review process that acts as an empowering tool and that also allows the group to enjoy its successes and to control the future.

Akira: I don't like the new social worker. By the time I get to know her you will be back. So, I don't think I'm going to bother getting to know her or come to group.

Christina: Like I've been saying, I'm gone when you're gone.

Zaria: I agree. Why bother if you're going to return? Why should we get to know someone when you're only coming back. That is, you're coming back, right?

Nancy: She said that she was coming back. Right?

John: (panicked) What? You're not coming back? You said you were!

PW: I'm coming back. The reason Doris is going to take over the group is because everyone has worked hard to build this group and I don't want to see it go by the wayside when I leave.

Akira: When you come back we will return too.

PW: I'm not sure why everyone is against attending the group while I'm gone.

Christina: It's just too hard to get to know someone new. We know everyone here and it's running so well. So, when you return it will be like nothing changed.

PW: Really? I'm not so sure.

Akira: I don't work well with others. Remember when you started and how distant I was?

PW: Yes, it took you a while to get to know me, but you did. How about anyone else? Can you remember back to when you began the group or program and had to get to know the staff?

Akira: Yeah, you scared me. You were so perky. (Akira does her imitation of the worker. The rest of the group members perform their imitations in return. The group has a good laugh.)

PW: Those were great imitations. Despite all your first impressions you all kept coming to the group and to the program for services. That is a wonderful ability you all have.

Nancy: I don't care what all you think. I've gone through many staff changes when I was at my old program and I'm going to keep coming no matter who is here. This group is important to me. It's the only safe place I can talk about what's going on with me.

Akira: Okay, maybe I will show up. It was just hard when Kathy left and there was no one to replace her. We were stuck at the program without a social worker for so long. I wasn't sure anyone was coming. It felt like the period after my father died. Alone.

As the discussion about the leave of absence and transfer continued within the group, the PW began to sense that the members were able to go deeper by connecting their current feelings to past experiences. It was just too easy to be angry at the PW and to dislike the IW. At this point the PW decided to remind them of the time when she was the new worker and their reactions toward her. Changing the focus provided them with an opportunity to make the connection between their initial reactions about the PW and their initial reactions to the new worker. Then, they were able to begin to explore their feelings and other situations with other agency personnel and family members that stimulated similar feelings of loss and abandonment.

As Malekoff (2004) states, "endings in adolescent groups cannot be taken for granted" (p. 186). He points out that the adolescents of today have already experienced a number of unceremonious separations throughout their short lives. Relationships with loved ones seem to come and go in a "revolving-door fashion." Therefore, adolescents need supportive environments to help them to work through the painful feelings generated by loss, and any termination/transfer process provides just such an opportunity. "There is an emergence of residual feelings that flow out of the echoes of past losses. A skilled group worker will use the termination stage of any group to help its members through an ending transition that is sensitive to these echoes, which can often go unheard and unanswered in the course of everyday life" (Malekoff, 2004, p. 186). In this group, many of the adolescent members reacted with statements of flight, deciding that they would leave before the PW left and IW began, illustrated in the continuous statement, "I'm gone when you're gone."

In the beginning, group members were reluctant to take a chance on the IW. As members began to talk about their feelings, however, they were able to connect to past experiences of losses. Malekoff (2004) states "Endings are likely to arouse powerful emotions and memories associated with past separations and losses" (p. 188). Time is always needed to process feelings, therefore, and to move through transitions sensitively and thoughtfully. An abrupt leave of absence not well facilitated can add to past losses and even hurt the relationship with the PW upon her return. Thus, the PW and IW both believed that it was best to leave the group with a sense of security, realizing that a poor transfer could also affect members' trust in the whole program.

By the due date the IW had taken over and was leading the group. The group had begun planning their knitting projects, and the IW had been able to establish a working relationship with the members. Thus, the PW was assured that the group would continue in her absence.

REINTRODUCING THE PRIMARY WORKER

Scheduling the PW's return needs to be determined as soon as possible. In this case, before the Primary Worker left the group was co-led to assist in the initial transition, and this process was also used to reintroduce the PW. Thus, the first group session that the PW attends should be co-led in order to give group members the opportunity to review what occurred during her absence and to allows the group time to say goodbye to the IW. After welcoming the PW back the group should once again participate in redefining goals, purpose, and direction. As in the case of the initial transfer, it is important to remember that no group can remain the same when there is a transfer of workers.

PW: It's great to be back with all of you. What happened while I was gone?

Akira: I made a couple funny looking scarves.

Christina: I just couldn't get the hang of knitting and I kept losing the needles.

Kim: I loved knitting. I made everyone scarves for Christmas!

PW: Lisa, Nancy, how was the knitting group for you?

Lisa: It gave me time to do lots of knitting. I'm working on a baby blanket for my son.

Nancy: I didn't even try knitting. I came though and we all still talked.

IW: I would like to take pictures with everyone . . . (group takes pictures).

PW: It looks as though the group was successful at learning to knit. (Group members give praise to Doris for teaching and assisting them in learning to knit.)

IW: It was great working with everyone in this group. I had a good time knitting and talking with all of you.

Akria: Where are the pictures of the baby? (The remainder of the meeting was spent looking at the baby pictures, asking questions about the birth, motherhood, and updating the PW on all the events that she had missed.)

Gradual reintroduction of the PW to the group allows members the time to assess what they have achieved during a leave of absence as well as time to separate from the IW. In this case, the PW experienced mixed emotions. On one hand she was excited to see that the group had remained active during her leave, but she also felt anxious because several new members had been permitted to join the group, although it was unclear if this group was appropriate for their particular needs and goals. Still, this meeting gave the PW a little time to get to know the new group members and to begin working on a new agreement and to review the purpose of the group, making the switch back from activity to support. At the same time, the PW was concerned that this switch might be difficult and awkward for new members, who did not know the goals and norms of the group when it was a discussion-oriented therapeutic support group. The PW then realized that it would have been useful to meet with the IW before this meeting in order to start with a better sense of the new group, including the new members. Such a meeting would have also reduced her anxiety over the nature of the relationships between new and continuing members.

CONCLUSION

The transfer process described here was successful in maintaining group attendance and participation because it was planned and thoughtful. The group experienced the ability to continue attending while working with a new worker, providing an opportunity for growth. They were able to experience an absence with someone who did return as promised, undoing past unpleasant experiences associated with termination and loss, and it was also an effective way for members to experience a transition from one leader to another.

This opportunity also served to help the group members realize that a group can help them to meet their needs and resolve problems. They did not come to the group just to please the worker or because they were mandated; they were in the group to care for themselves and for one another, developing a supportive network regardless of the change in worker. In fact, the thought that went into the transition from one worker to another may even have made them stronger as individuals and closer as a group.

Further, this leave of absence provided a unique opportunity for the PW to model the importance of self care. By learning that they could take care of themselves and one another, the pervasive and potent power of mutual aid helped them through a challenging time (Steinberg, 2004).

Finally, both workers learned how important it is to develop a comprehensive transfer process with ample time for the transferring leadership and open dialogue. Workers must have time to plan and collaborate around transfer. Members must have time to express their fears and concerns, must be allowed to be part of the process, and must become invested in the transfer and its outcome. When that happens, when careful planning and collaboration are part of a transfer, this difficult process can provide opportunities for personal and interpersonal growth.

REFERENCES

Brandler, S. and Roman, C. (1999). *Group work: Skills and strategies for effective interventions*. Binghamton, New York: The Haworth Press, Inc.

Kurland, R. and Salmon, R. (1998). *Teaching a methods course in social work with groups*. Alexandria, VA: Council on Social Work Education.

Mackenzie, K. (1996). Time limited group psychotherapy. *International Journal of Group Psychotherapy*, (26), 41-60.

Maholick, L. and Turner, D. (1997). Termination: That difficult farewell. *American Journal of Psychotherapy*, (33), 583-591.

Malekoff, A. (2004). *Group work with adolescents: Principles and practice*. New York: Guilford Press.

McGee, T. (1974). Therapist termination in group psychotherapy. *International Journal of Group Psychotherapy*, (24), 3-12.

Northen, H. and Kurland, R. (2001). *Social work with groups.* New York: Columbia University Press.

Siebold, C. (1991). When the therapist leaves. *Clinical Social Work Journal*, (19), 191-204.

Steinberg, D. (2004). *The mutual-aid approach to working with groups: Helping people help one another.* Binghamton, New York: The Haworth Press, Inc.

Vichnis, R. (1999). Passing the baton: Principles and implications for transferring leadership of a group. *Social Work with Groups*, 22(2/3), 139-158.

Yalom, I. (1995). *The theory and practice of group psychotherapy.* New York: Harper Collins.

A Worker's Personal Grief and Its Impact on Processing a Group's Termination

Camille P. Roman

SUMMARY. This article deals with a worker struggling with a personal loss while simultaneously helping her group with the termination of a valued long term member. The focus is on the parallel grieving process and the resistance to mourning. *[Article copies available for a fee from The Haworth Document Delivery Service: 1-800-HAWORTH. E-mail address: <docdelivery@haworthpress.com> Website: <http://www.HaworthPress.com> © 2006 by The Haworth Press, Inc. All rights reserved.]*

KEYWORDS. Group termination, stages of group development, worker's personal loss, grief, parallel process

I have of late been thinking about beginning again after loss, and grief. This is not surprising to me since my sister died recently and shortly thereafter my friend died. While struggling with the multitude of feelings that come and go when one experiences loss, I continued to work with a group that has been together for ten years. One evening a long term group member announced that she would be moving to Israel

---

The author offers special thanks to her dear friend, Dr. Sondra Brandler, and her beloved mentor, Dr. Robert Salmon.

This article is dedicated to the author's sister Phyllis.

[Haworth co-indexing entry note]: "A Worker's Personal Grief and Its Impact on Processing a Group's Termination." Roman, Camille P. Co-published simultaneously in *Social Work with Groups* (The Haworth Press, Inc.) Vol. 29, No. 2/3, 2006, pp. 235-242; and: *Making Joyful Noise: The Art, Science, and Soul of Group Work* (ed: Andrew Malekoff, Robert Salmon, and Dominique Moyse Steinberg) The Haworth Press, Inc., 2006, pp. 235-242. Single or multiple copies of this article are available for a fee from The Haworth Document Delivery Service [1-800-HAWORTH, 9:00 a.m. - 5:00 p.m. (EST). E-mail address: docdelivery@haworthpress.com].

and thus leaving the group. With that announcement, we all entered the termination stage, and, for me, I felt the professional boundary between myself and the group becoming more porous.

Prior to that evening, my work offered me respite from a seemingly endless stream of difficult feelings. Up until that night, I was able to compartmentalize my grief and my work effectively, or so I thought. I was soon to discover how much of my "self" had been absent from my work and therefore how ineffective I really was during this period. The group was not about to allow me to continue to separate myself out and consequently, it forced me to deal with my loss more honestly.

I would like to share with you my thoughts about this struggle: a worker and her group trying to move forward while confronting the complexities of loss. In this discussion I will look at the parallel process of loss between a long term group whose member is leaving and the worker who has experienced the recent death of a sibling. I will attempt to show how the predictable process specific to the termination stage offers a structure of safety to both worker and group, enabling them to process this most difficult period. I also intend that this discussion will show how the individual stages of grieving correspond to the issues in the termination stage of a group.

I hope these thoughts will be healing to me in my journey and informative to you in yours, since I know well it is a voyage we all must take. The very nature of our work demands that we deal with the always threatening collision between the worker's personal struggles and the group's work. Termination triggers the ". . . pain of loss and endings that stalks all of us, worker and client alike . . ." (Brandler and Roman, 1999, p. 94). Old issues of separation and individuation are reactivated for worker and group, making the processing of this stage potentially very difficult.

In Brandler and Roman (1999) the reader is asked to think of the group as a separate living entity, ". . . a being with its own personality composed of many separate and unique parts each part contributing to the whole . . . It has a total personality . . . distinct from any other." The authors suggest that like an individual that is multifaceted, the "conflicting components within the complex structure struggle against each other towards resolution and growth" (Brandler and Roman, 1999, p. 321). This challenge and subsequent resolution of conflict results in a "healthier" being. Thus, the group as a whole begins at a primitive level of functioning and ends at a more developed level. Ideally, the group ends when maximum growth is achieved or its goals are reached.

The end of a group is the end of a life. In a group where there is a high level of intimacy established over time through mutual struggle and built on a strong cohesive base, the leaving of a member is like a death in the family. Whether it is a group ending or an individual member leaving, when a termination occurs, a mourning phase is initiated and a grieving process begins (Shulman, 1979). "In all groups, while the particulars may vary, the letting go is difficult for worker and clients. For both, termination triggers memories of unresolved endings and accompanying loss" (Brandler and Roman, 1999, p. 11).

These residual historical losses can contaminate the group's ability to grieve effectively. If this occurs, the mourning is incomplete and the members' abilities to move forward establishing new intimate relationships will be compromised. For this reason, the worker needs to be keenly aware of her personal feelings and the tasks she must address in her role as worker in helping the group process through the termination phase.

One of the primary tasks of the worker during the ending stage of the group is to help identify and consolidate gains. The identification of achievements and the validation of progress enable the group to make conscious its strengths and experience a sense of mastery and growth. This process takes place through a thorough evaluation of the group's experience. Reminiscing and sharing memories, both positive and negative, reinforces the cohesive group bond. Re-establishing a solid base enables members to then express any ambivalent feelings or unresolved conflicts. The worker's task is to enable the group to verbalize these complex feelings, accept them, and subsequently accept any feelings of helplessness and resignation associated with "unfinished business" (Kurland and Salmon, 1998). The worker needs to be, and needs to help the group to be sensitive to members who struggle with feelings of regret and loss. The nonjudgmental acceptance of these difficult feelings helps normalize them and allows members to move ahead and not get stuck in what could or should have been. The worker must help the group confront the inevitability of change and our powerlessness to stop it. Simultaneously the worker moves to focus the group forward reinforcing gains, and the ability to achieve in the next arena. The task for all is to integrate strengths, accept limits, and advance. This can be a difficult process as it was for me in my work with a long term group.

I am feeling comfortable in group during the evening of Malka's disclosure. The group is talking about their difficulty confronting painful decisions. Malka suddenly says, "Speaking of confronting difficult decisions, I'm struggling all night with my mixed feelings about telling you all that my husband and I have decided to move to Israel." The group reacts with surprise and disbelief. Malka had mentioned her moving as an outside chance several months ago. The group and I had not followed up on this matter (did not want to know?), and so her decision feels sudden and totally unexpected.

I feel a surge of anger. "What is she talking about," I yell in my head, "she can't leave now, she is not 'ready' and besides she didn't even let us know." Various members express disbelief and denial. Beatrice insists Malka could call in for our sessions. Terri laughs and expresses feelings of betrayal. Susan comments that she knew sooner or later someone would leave and she is sorry she had ever joined the group.

That night after leaving the group I feel exhausted. I prefer to attribute my weariness to the lack of sleep rather than my psychic struggle to repress my overwhelming feelings.

The next few weeks feel unproductive. Members come late more often, absences increase and I keep starting the group late because of one unexpected problem or another. Old conflicts resurface. Beatrice and Terri resume an old interactive pattern of attacking and competing. Susan withdraws by interacting less or talking about concrete problems rather than substantive emotional issues. Selma is angry most of the time and Maria is always 'nice' and non-confrontational, taking few emotional risks as she had behaved long ago. I feel more frustrated and unenthusiastic. Cognitively I know I am off but emotionally I am drained.

One night while I am preparing for group I think to myself, "ugh, more termination anguish tonight!" For the first time in weeks, I hear myself. I am reacting to the loss of the group members as if she were my sister. I was not prepared for my sister's death, although I knew it was coming. I wasn't "ready" to let her go. I am angry that I have to experience the loss. I don't want to feel her absence in my life. Most of all I feel powerless; I can do nothing.

When Malka announced her leaving, I, like the group, felt unprepared. We were not "ready" to lose a wonderful rich relationship. We wanted to deny it would happen ("she can call in from Israel"). We were angry that there was nothing we could do to stop her ("can you postpone this?"). I began to distance as did the group. Our coming late, not talking honestly and openly about feelings and our withdrawing emotionally were all expressions of the fear and anxiety we associated with the loss of a significant person.

I suddenly saw this regressive behavior as being a "normal" part of a group's and an individual's reaction to loss. Often when we are confronted with the irretrievable we revert to a more familiar, psychically safe place, old behavior: Selma's old angry defense, Maria's old "nice guy" routine (as the group had labeled it earlier), Susan's old withdrawal ("the lone ranger" as members had affectionately described her), and the intense old sibling rivalry characteristic of the relationship between Beatrice and Terri.

There it all was clearly before me–the termination stage. I couldn't see it before because the historical noise of my chaotic childhood forced me into hiding. That childhood, filled with multiple losses, has resurfaced during my sister's dying. As I was faced with an unbearable loss, my old defenses kicked in. The past was all too present and was stopping me for going forward. As I was stuck, so too was the group (Kurland and Salmon, 1993).

Once I saw what was happening I was able to feel an element of safety again in the predictable structure of the termination stage. Characteristic responses during the termination stage are: denial (you can call in), regression (old sibling rivalry behavior), flight (increase in my lateness), anxiety and regret (I should have never joined), and withdrawal (not speaking of feelings). It now made sense. Cognitive understanding provided me with a framework for my feelings thus giving them less power and allowing me to use the feelings, therapeutically (Ormont, 2001).

How interesting, I mused, the process of my breaking through this countertransferential block was a living example of something I often speak about to students. When discussing the use of self as a therapeutic tool, I lecture that the worker must feel free to immerse herself in her feelings. The challenge is to feel and let those feelings pass through a cognitive filter that enables distance from the feeling and insight into its connection to the group's process. The fear of most workers is that you can get lost in your feelings and become ineffectual. I had forgotten "the impulse to protect the self and not allow the group to go where it needs to go in order to do its work is strong. The group must be held to the work, no matter how frightening it is for the worker" (Roman, 2002,

p. 63). I had come close. I must share this with my class but for now I had work to do. I had to reclaim the worker's role in the ending stage of group development (Kurland and Salmon, 1998, pp. 218-219). This would serve to help the group, and me.

The following evening I am on time for group. Members trickle in with a variety of explanations for arriving late. I comment that recently it seems difficult for us to start on time. Selma rolls her eyes, and suggests that "life is complicated. You can't predict what's going to happen, schedule changes, problems with the kids–you know." I hear the latent message–it is complicated here, we can't control things and we're not sure we're up to confronting it. I pursue, "How else are things complicated?" Selma leads the charge, "Oh, here she goes! What's that supposed to mean?" "Yeah and how do you 'feel' about those complications," Terri mocks. We all laugh.

This group has been here before, struggling to risk. I say, "You know I agree with your analysis Selma. Things are complicated and unpredictable and it's exhausting trying to still be here. We've all been running scared lately, including me. I've been starting late for weeks." "Yeah, I wanted to say something," Malka comments, "it's unusual for you and everyone to come late but I felt since I was leaving it wasn't my place anymore to say anything." "You think there is some connection here between my behavior, the group's behavior and Malka's leaving?" I inquire. They agree there may be some connection.

Maria replies that she has also been disappointed in the return of her "nice guy" attitude and her old inability to say she was annoyed with not only the lateness but also the superficial level of discussion. Terri comments, "Yeah and I noticed the return of the 'Lone Ranger'" referring to Susan's old pattern of withdrawal. We laugh, relieved to be present again with each other. Selma is quick to pick up on Terri's comment. Looking at me, Selma quips, "You also were rather 'quiet.' " I own up to my avoidant behavior and share with them my analysis of what had happened. And with a "hearty high ho Silver," we are off and running. I have finally given permission for the group to express their honest feelings, by being honest myself. We are again bonded and safe enough to risk.

They verbalize, with great gusto, their anger at Malka for leaving and me for abandoning them when I was most needed. They talk about their guilt; how could they be angry with me, my sister had died. All of these women have suffered the loss of an intimate other; they know I must be in pain. At the same time, they struggle with feelings of resentment at having to "take care of me," by denying their own pain. Terri proclaims her lack of empathy for me. She needs to hold on to her anger. They all have functioned as "parentified" children in their families. Fear of loss, anger, resentment, sorrow and compassion fill the room for ninety minutes. I marvel at their insights, honesty and at their ability to own their group.

We had broken through the fear. I went home feeling exhausted and elated at the same time. What a group! We had done good work. For the first time in weeks I slept soundly.

We are still processing the loss of Malka and what that represents to us. Some sessions are more intense than others. My feelings of loss were further intensified by the loss of a colleague and friend some months later, but the group did not know about that and was already deep into their work. I felt the old sense of sadness and the impulse to withdraw but the group was so present, they would not allow it. They demanded my presence by being active and confrontational. I had recovered my professional distance and my ability to be empathic without merging. I was able to reclaim, and resume the worker's role, as needed, in helping the group deal with loss and endings.

Both the group and I went into mourning when each was confronted with the loss of a significant relationship. Our grief processes paralleled. Individual grieving and group grieving are both characterized by denial, anger, withdrawal, bargaining, depression, and finally acceptance (Kubler-Ross, 1969; Northen and Kurland, 2001). When I was able to identify how my own mourning reflected the mourning of the group, I was able to connect the two. The use of a model for the termination phase enabled me to process the feelings in the safety of a cognitive structure (Kurland and Salmon, 1998, pp. 218-219).

Both worker and group continue to work on building new relationships, acknowledging the contribution of those gone, and accepting the totality of our feelings. We have again experienced what Carl Jung said so eloquently, that "One does not become enlightened by imagining light but by making darkness conscious" (Zweig and Abraham, 1990, p. 4).

REFERENCES

Brandler, S. and Roman, C.P. (1999). *Group work: Skills and strategies for effective interventions.* 2nd edition, New York: The Haworth Press, Inc.

Jung, Carl as quoted in Zweig, C. and Abraham, J. (1990). *Meeting the shadow: The hidden power of the dark side of human nature.* New York: Penguin Putnam, 4.

Kubler-Ross, E. (1969). *On death and dying.* New York: Macmillan Publishing Co., Inc.

Kurland, R. and Salmon, R. (1998). *Teaching a methods course in social group work with groups.* Alexandria, VA: Council on Social Work Education.

Kurland, R. and Salmon, R. (1993). Not just one of the gang: Group workers and their role as an authority. *Social Work with Groups,* 16 (1/2), 153-167.

Northen, H. and Kurland, R. (2001). *Social work with groups,* 3rd edition, New York: Columbia University Press.

Ormont, L. (2001). Training group therapists through the study of countertransferences. In Lena B. Furger (ed.), *The technique of group treatment.* CT: Psychosocial Press, 175-189.

Roman, C.P. (2002). It's not always easy to sit on your mouth, *Social Work with Groups,* 25 (1/2), 61-64.

Yalom, I. (1995). *Theory and practice of group psychotherapy.* 3rd edition, USA.: Basic Books.

Caregiver Support Groups: Finding Common Ground

Helene Ebenstein

SUMMARY. Members of caregiver support groups for the elderly have much in common but also bring to the group different experiences and attitudes. This article explores how group workers knowledgeable about significant caregiver differences and their effects on the group can enrich the group experience for all members. The four caregiver issues examined are: (1) past history between the caregiver and care recipient, (2) ability of caregiver to privately pay for home care, (3) views on long-term care placement in a nursing home, and (4) stage of disease or level of care needed by care recipient. Essential beliefs regarding the value of differences described by Northen and Kurland provide a framework for the group worker. *[Article copies available for a fee from The Haworth Document Delivery Service: 1-800-HAWORTH. E-mail address: <docdelivery@haworthpress.com> Website: <http://www.HaworthPress.com> © 2006 by The Haworth Press, Inc. All rights reserved.]*

KEYWORDS. Caregiver support groups, common ground, conflict, differences, family caregivers, group work

INTRODUCTION

Family caregivers of the elderly share many concerns but they are also a heterogeneous group in many ways. As they come together in

[Haworth co-indexing entry note]: "Caregiver Support Groups: Finding Common Ground." Ebenstein, Helene. Co-published simultaneously in *Social Work with Groups* (The Haworth Press, Inc.) Vol. 29, No. 2/3, 2006, pp. 243-258; and: *Making Joyful Noise: The Art, Science, and Soul of Group Work* (ed: Andrew Malekoff, Robert Salmon, and Dominique Moyse Steinberg) The Haworth Press, Inc., 2006, pp. 243-258. Single or multiple copies of this article are available for a fee from The Haworth Document Delivery Service [1-800-HAWORTH, 9:00 a.m. - 5:00 p.m. (EST). E-mail address: docdelivery@haworthpress.com].

doi:10.1300/J009v29n02_16

caregiver support groups, the challenge for group workers is to help members with differing viewpoints and experiences find common ground. Caregiver support group members talk of the comfort of realizing that they are not alone. They see everyone in the room going through similar experiences and truly understanding how it feels to be a caregiver (Toseland, 1995). But that essential feeling of group support can be strained by potentially divisive differences among members.

Although it may appear preferable to recruit support group members who share as many characteristics as possible, that is usually not feasible as potential members are not standing in line. Homogeneity may not even be the best approach (Bertcher and Maple, 1985). A more diverse membership offers more opportunity for rethinking long held beliefs and considering new options. Northen and Kurland (2001) provide invaluable guidance to workers on the importance of differences. They discuss how differences can contribute to the richness of the group; that looking at differences benefits all; that disagreeing is not synonymous with disliking; and expressing differences will not tear the group apart. Bolstered by these essential beliefs regarding differences, group workers who are also knowledgeable about the issues which can cause conflict among caregivers are ready when differences surface. They are in a better position to help the group accept these differences and use them to foster mutual aid (Steinberg, 2004).

This paper will discuss four commonly encountered caregiver issues which can affect both the early and middle stages of caregiver support groups by threatening group bonding and by creating rifts among group members (Kurland and Salmon, 1998; Northen and Kurland, 2001; Kelly and Berman-Rossi, 1999). These issues are: past history between the caregiver and the care recipient, ability of caregiver to privately pay for home care, views on long-term placement in a nursing home, and stage of disease or level of care needed by the care recipient. The intent of the discussion is to prepare workers by exploring the differing viewpoints and experiences of members regarding these issues as well as highlighting the effects they may have on the group as a whole. Worker strategies for retaining new members and using reactions to differences to the group's advantage will also be covered. The essential beliefs about differences described by Northen and Kurland (2001) will be used as a framework. Examples of group process from the caregiver support group facilitated by the author will illustrate how a group deals with the issues and include the worker's successful as well as off base interventions.

The skyrocketing increase in the number of family caregivers has already made the need for programs and services for this population a priority. National surveys estimate that one in four households contains a family caregiver. Close to 30 million people are now providing some long-term care to a family member or friend. Their unpaid care is estimated to be worth between $275 and $300 billion annually (Polivka, 2005). The increase is fueled by the rapidly rising number of those age 85 and older (Mui and Burnette, 1994). This group is most likely to require the help of family members as they are living with chronic illnesses, are discharged earlier from hospitals and rely more on outpatient care (Houts, Nezu, Nezu, and Bucher, 1996). The toll on family caregivers is high. They often feel burdened and depressed (Fredman and Daly, 1998; The Henry J. Kaiser Family Foundation, 2002) and have many physical problems (Schulz, O'Brien, Bookwala, and Fleissner, 1995). Caregivers also suffer economically as they work part-time or leave the workforce completely (Feder, Komisar, and Niefeld, 2000). Despite the pressures, many caregivers find great satisfaction in the work they do and are grateful that they can be there for a family member.

CAREGIVER SUPPORT GROUPS

The large and ever growing number of caregivers has sparked the relatively new specialty of family caregiver services. Social workers play key roles in programs designed to provide information, education and emotional support to family caregivers. Support groups are often included in the array of services. Typically, support group goals include releasing emotions, validating concerns, reducing social isolation, obtaining information, improving coping, decreasing stress, and problem-solving. Members share their experiences, provide information, give advice and draw out other members (Galinsky and Shopler, 1995). Toseland (1995) clarifies that support group members expect to receive support, not "therapy." Workers focus on developing a climate of trust, empathy, warmth and cohesion.

Caregiver support groups are frequently ongoing, long-term groups, serving as a resource over an often very lengthy caregiving career (McCallion and Toseland, 1995). For the past five years, the author has led such a group for adult children caring for a parent with dementia. Bi-weekly meetings take place in a large hospital in Manhattan. Currently there are eight regularly attending group members whose parents are in the middle or late stages of their illness. The group is evenly divided by gender and ethnically diverse. Members run the gamut regarding living and home care arrangements. The goals of the group are to provide mutual support, exchange information, and improve coping and caregiving skills. Group composition changes as members leave when parents die and new members join. The ongoing nature of the group blurs the boundaries of group stages. Every nine months or so, a long-time member may leave the group and/or a new member joins. The members and worker are adjusting to beginnings, middles, and ends throughout the year (Kurland and Salmon, 1998; Northen and Kurland, 2001; Kelly and Berman-Rossi, 1999). Although some caregiver support groups have closed membership and are time-limited, many operate as describe above.

PAST HISTORY BETWEEN CAREGIVER
AND CARE RECIPIENT

Roberta Satow (2005) writes "But after a lifetime of being angry at my mother for not taking care of me, I find myself in a position for which I am not prepared–having to take care of *her*" (p. 9). Although many caregivers may have trouble expressing such feelings, they are in similar situations. In order for them to bond with group members, they must be able to talk about their troubled relationship with a family member without feeling judged and criticized. Group members who idealize the relationship they had with the person for whom they are caring will be challenged to listen to another person's experience without judging themselves the better caregiver. It is important for the group to deal with this issue both in the beginning and middle stages. A new member who believes he/she is the only person in the group with a difficult past history will not remain a group member. During the middle stage, when members are more open and trusting, there is opportunity for all members to enrich their understanding of the complexities of relationships and accept the inevitability of conflicting emotions regarding caregiving.

The group worker's handling of this issue is key. First, it is important that the worker be aware of his/her own feelings about who is a good caregiver as this will be helpful in understanding the reactions of group members and prevent subtly siding with a preferred type of caregiver. Encouraging members to talk more openly about their past relationships with care recipients, remembering both the positive and the negative, will help to highlight the many facets of all relationships and normalize conflicting feelings. Stereotypes will fade as members reach across the divide to understand more fully what it is like for caregivers who have had very different relationships. Perhaps all group members can begin to recognize the courage and strength needed "to do right thing" even when there is no love. They can also appreciate the efforts of caregivers who wish to honor and repay a relative for all that has been given. The ability to empathize despite differences is vital to promoting mutual respect and aid. The "good" caregiver may have the chance to ease the burden of maintaining an ideal relationship and the "bad" caregiver may nurture a stronger bond with a family member. Despite differences in past histories, many caregiver experiences are similar. Instead of vying with each other, the worker helps the group to recognize the universal feelings and emotions of caregiving and to normalize them. Incorporating the view of Northen and Kurland (2001) that continuing discussion of this issue enriches the group and benefits all helps clear the path for the worker. If the issue is not being discussed, it is likely simmering beneath the surface. The worker's task is to model the process of mutual aid by raising taboo issues if useful and no one else is (Steinberg, 2004) while keeping in mind that members are expecting support not therapy.

The following example occurred in the support group for adult children caring for a parent with dementia. Since this is a long-term group, when parents die caregivers drop out and new members join an already established group. This arrangement complicates the workers job of gauging the stage of the group.

Sonia, a 63-year-old only child caring for her mother, was attending her first group meeting. Towards the end of the group, the following interchange occurred.

> Nora: My mother and I have always been best friends. She is the most important person in my life and always has been. That is why it is so terrible for me to see her go downhill. When I think about the future I get scared and depressed. But I'm determined to always be there for her and I'm glad that I can do that.

> Sonia: I don't know if I'll feel comfortable in this group. Everyone here is very close to their parent but my mother and I were never like that. My mother was always very cold and critical and either we fought a lot or didn't have much to do with each other. She needs me now and I'm taking care of her because I can't turn my back on her. She is still my mother and I guess I love her.

Robert: I think you can learn a lot here. People come in with all kinds of good information. The more people, the more you can learn.

Other group members shake their heads in agreement.

There is silence.

Group worker: Robert, I agree. You can get a lot of useful information here but (looking at the group) is Sonia correct? Did everyone in the group have a close relationship with their parent?

There is silence.

In this illustration, Nora was linking her suffering with the close relationship she always had with her mother. The implication is that it is easier if your relationship has not been close. Sonia bravely expressed her discomfort at being different from the perceived group norm. Many new members would have said nothing and not returned. Robert, who actually had a tumultuous history with his parents, tried to encourage and welcome her but did not address her discomfort. The group worker was attempting to reassure Sonia by creating an opportunity for members to talk about their difficult relationships with a parent. This was not appropriate. Although other members knew each other, they did not know Sonia and may not have been comfortable talking so soon about their troubled family histories. A better approach would have been to focus on the many shared experiences and feelings that all group members were having. This would have helped reassure Sonia that she had much in common with the members and would get something more from the meetings than information. Sonia did continue as a member despite the bumpy first meeting and helped other members speak more honestly about problems they had with a parent.

ABILITY OF FAMILY TO PAY FOR HOME CARE

Many caregiver support groups are not homogenous in terms of class and income level. Members often range from the wealthy to those who wonder how they will pay the rent. What effect do these differences have on the group's ability to bond and empathize with each other? The impact can play itself out in interesting ways, some of them unexpected to an unwary group worker. Home attendant care is one of the most discussed issues in caregiver support groups. Members provide feedback about the need for a home care worker and are likely to have much information and experience about the process which they are eager to share. In addition to the significant practical concerns, there are intense emotional reactions to the use of paid home care. Feelings of failure, guilt, grief over the continuing deterioration, fear of the future and conflicts with family members are just some of the issues. These factors create problems between members who are dependent on Medicaid or other subsidized home care programs and those who hire and privately pay for homecare.

Group members who depend on Medicaid or other subsidized programs bemoan the system, the constant replacement of home care workers, the poor quality of the home care received, the struggle to get additional hours and the unresponsiveness of administrators. They express frustration at perceived lack of control, worry about the care a family member is receiving and fear sudden reductions in service due to budget cuts. It may be difficult for a member in this position to empathize with the problems of a caregiver who can get the best help, hire and fire at will, and pay for as much care as is needed. Despite their privileged position, however, these members still seem to complain and worry too. To complicate things further, many caregivers who are neither wealthy nor poor, are paying for home care. Resentful that others are receiving this care for free, they complain that their family member has worked all their life but is not entitled to Medicaid although their savings are not nearly enough to pay for the care they need. Parents spend their life savings and caregivers sometimes endanger their financial futures by using their funds. These members feel that the wealthy and poor can get needed home care but the middle class is getting a raw deal.

The group is a microcosm reflecting the larger cultural and economic pressures that pit people against each other in the world (Gearing, 2002). What can the worker do to help the group deal with these very real and understandable feelings and reactions? The advice given by Kurland and Salmon (1997) regarding group norms are applicable here. "Through modeling, supporting, limiting, and teaching, it is the worker who has a major influence." The worker models by bringing the issue to the surface if that has not happened and encouraging open discussion of the differing experiences of group members. She supports by validating the reactions and feelings even when their expression may cause discomfort among members. If members begin to attack each other or scapegoat, the worker limits that type of behavior and models a style that continues discussion in a more tolerant environment. Members will learn that nearly every caregiver, regardless of financial situation, dreads the need for home care, worries about its quality, mourns the decline of a family member and tries to gain control of an uncontrollable situation. The worker teaches that group members are actually "all in the same boat" in many significant ways while at the same time acknowledging the very real differences in experiences. All group members benefit and learn that expressing differences will not destroy the group but will actually strengthen it.

The following example occurred in the support group for adult children caring for a parent with dementia.

> Harriet: I am having such a hard time getting my mother's home attendant to stop doing everything for her. I keep telling her that if my mother can still do something she should let her. I fill the house with my mother's favorite foods so they can cook together. But when I go downstairs, I see my mother just sitting while the home attendant cooks.

> Alma: You can work with the same person. With my mother, I never know who they will be sending next. In the last month, Medicaid has sent five different people and I'm afraid to complain because they might cut me off.

> A few other members shake their head in understanding.

> Bonnie: You can call the supervisor at the home care agency. Maybe that will help.

> Worker: I think Alma may be raising another issue. Do some members feel that Harriet has less to worry about because she can privately hire her own home attendant?

> Alma: I feel that way. I wish I had a two family house and could move my mother to the ground floor apartment like Harriet did. That would make things so much easier for me. Also, when you're paying, you're in charge. You're the boss.

> Harriet: You know, it's funny. I'm watching my mother go downhill and I'm trying to do everything I can think of to help her but in the end there is nothing that I can do. It's out of my control. I never thought that anyone would think I'm the lucky one but it's true, I have it a lot better than some other people.

Alma leans over and touches Harriet's shoulder: I know that you are going through a lot too. I didn't mean to make you feel bad.

Worker: Talking about what's on your minds is a good thing. It will help you understand each other better and get closer.

In this situation, there is an undercurrent in Alma's response and the body language of other group members implying that Harriet does not have the right to complain. Her worries are not as significant as Alma's. When Bonnie responds to Alma's particular problem, the group begins to glide away from a potentially divisive issue that is just below the surface. The worker brings the group back by framing what Alma is saying, thereby encouraging the members to speak more openly. The worker models this behavior showing that the group can discuss the issue. Harriet's response begins what should become an ongoing exploration of the members' feelings on this topic. A group norm is being reinforced–it is possible to talk openly about sensitive issues without attacking members and disagreeing is not synonymous with disliking.

VIEWS ON LONG-TERM PLACEMENT IN A NURSING HOME

The image of a heartless family member abandoning a relative for placement in a nursing home haunts many caregivers. Caregivers are admired as long as their relative remains at home. Sometimes adding to the pressure are promises made or pleas from parents or spouses to "never put me in a nursing home." The effect on most caregivers is to do everything possible to continue care at home. Generally, caregivers who join a support group do have their relative at home. Over time the situation usually worsens and some caregivers feel they simply cannot go on. How do the worker and the group help members cope with an overwhelming situation and allow discussion of nursing home placement without stigmatizing those who might be considering it? Without help from the worker, the issue may be taboo, with members choosing to leave the group rather than risk feeling ostracized for even considering placement. Returning to the essential beliefs regarding conflict described by Northen and Kurland (2001) assures the worker that the issue must be raised if it is not being discussed and that all will benefit from a frank exchange of views. Kurland and Salmon (1997) provide a blueprint for action by exhorting the worker to model, support, limit, and teach.

The worker's awareness of his/her own views on nursing home placement is necessary. The worker must constantly check her own impulses to point out ways that using a community resource might help keep a relative home a little longer. Knowledge of resources is vital but overemphasis can make it even more difficult for a member to choose placement. Encouraging discussion helps to normalize it as an option, gives members a chance to hear other viewpoints and may even lead to reconsidering firmly held opinions. Understanding why a member with whom you empathize might choose placement, lessens the instinct to criticize and judge. Those opposed to placement may feel they have permission to loosen the bonds of their own promises and commitments. Surprisingly, sometimes members who have placed relatives see them flourishing as they socialize with residents and staff and participate in activities. When this highly charged topic is aired, discussed and more fully understood, it ceases to be a touchstone for judging the worth of a caregiver. Long-term groups with changing membership are especially valuable in helping members expand their understanding of nursing home placement. They have the opportunity of seeing others make the decision to place a relative and act as models in this area. Members learn that placing a relative does not end the responsibility of caregiving. Many people visit regularly and continue to closely monitor care. They may also observe members who previously vetoed any possibility of considering placement begin to change their views. Although most caregivers do not place a relative in a nursing home, this option should not be rejected out of guilt, shame, and pressure.

The following example took place in the support group for adult children caring for a parent with dementia.

> Worker: Nora, you haven't been here in a while. What's been happening?

> Nora: Things have been terrible. My mother fell and broke her hip and I stayed with her 24/7 in the hospital and in the nursing home where she went for therapy. I never let her out of my sight. Things are so bad in nursing homes. The care is terrible and patients get ignored. Thank God my mother is back home.

> Alfred: You're right. For a time I was thinking about placing my mother in a home and I went to visit a few. But I just can't do it. It wouldn't make me feel better. I'd be worrying all the time. At least

when she's home with me she gets good care even though my whole life has been on hold for the last six years.

Worker: A few of you have parents in nursing homes and are looking uncomfortable. What's on your minds now?

Mary: I feel like running out of this room and getting to the nursing home to make sure my mother is OK.

Robert: I worry all the time too but I felt I had no choice. My mother didn't have a home to go back to.

Mary: I have to work and I kept missing time or rushing back from work afraid of what I would find. My mother wasn't eating and was sitting in the dark to save money. My life is much better and my mother has made some friends and is gaining weight.

Nora: For me that would never be an option. I'm going to be there with my mother as long as I'm around but I understand that everyone has to make their own decision.

Mary: I believe that I made the right decision. It's the only way that I can have any kind of balance in my life.

Ellen: Mary, what you said about your mother making friends makes me wonder if I'm doing the right thing for my father. He is so lonely in my apartment. Sometimes I think he might be happier being with other people.

In this example, Nora was expressing the very real and serious problems with hospital and nursing home care but also implying that the only place a relative is safe is at home. As Alfred agreed, the worker read the body language of a few members and encouraged them to express their views. The worker's action helped to set limits on a potentially one-sided view of nursing home problems, allowing Mary to acknowledge her fears and justify her decision to place. The result was an exchange of views and which gave Ellen a chance to think about placement a little differently.

STAGE OF DISEASE OR LEVEL OF CARE NEEDED BY CARE RECIPIENT

Who suffers more? Is it the caregiver plagued by a relative with dementia who repeats the same question incessantly or is it the caregiver of a relative who can no longer speak? If the goals of the group are to provide mutual support, exchange information and improve coping and caregiving skills, the focus on this question is misplaced. The worker's task here is to help move the group in a more productive direction while acknowledging the pain of each group member.

Regardless of the stage of the disease, members are dealing with loss, grief, fear, guilt, anger, and resentment. They can help each other and themselves by being encouraged to express those feelings and emotions and a host of others. For caregivers of relatives with most dementias there is no cure. Caregivers share that burden along with the frustration of lack of control. In the most important ways, members are "in the same boat" and the worker's job is to help members recognize this and support each other (Steinberg, 2004). Tensions among group members on this issue may also affect retention of new group members who are often caring for a relative in an earlier stage of illness. It is frightening enough to begin hearing about the future that lays ahead for a relative. To be viewed as someone who has nothing to complain about, would discourage even the most determined new member. Exchanging information is also vital to this issue. There are strategies for dealing with the difficult behavior of dementia and other illnesses. Members, especially those who have been through this, are in the best position to make suggestions about what works and what does not. Instead of competing about who is worse off, members not only support each other but may help reduce stressful situations. A knowledgeable worker can also provide invaluable information about techniques and strategies and recommend relevant books and articles. The worker is also needed to educate caregivers about the effects of illnesses and clarify that a relative is not intentionally behaving in a difficult way. A worker who is confident that openly discussing the problem will benefit all and that the members are capable of helping and learning from each other, will help the group tackle this issue and be strengthened.

The following is an example from the support group for adult children caring for a parent with dementia. Margaret is attending her second meeting.

Margaret: My father is still living on his own but things are really going downhill. I visit at least twice a week but I dread going there.

Sarah: You have to enjoy every day with him while he's still doing well. My mother doesn't get out of bed much anymore. I wish she could do half of the things your father is doing.

Alfred: When you're living with your parent there's no getting away. My mother is driving me nuts. She keeps hiding things to keep them safe and when she can't find them she says I stole them. We spent a few hours today looking for her dentures and I finally found them in the microwave. When I took them out my mother said she always knew they were there.

Worker: What's going on here?

Margaret: I don't know but I feel guilty for taking up the group's time when other people have it much worse than I do.

Sarah: I guess when I told you to enjoy every day I was talking about myself. I was so impatient with my mother at the beginning and I regret that. I don't want you to feel that way.

Margaret: But that's just one more thing for me to worry about. Whatever problems I have just don't seem as bad as every one else's but I'm a mess. How can I enjoy every day?

There is silence.

Worker: What do other people think? Do some people have it harder than others? Should you be counting your blessings if your parent is still able to live alone?

A few members look uncomfortable. After some moments of silence . . .

Robert: None of that matters. It's hard from day one and it never gets easy.

In this excerpt, it seems as if members are trying to top each other about who has it worse. This leaves the newest member, whose father is in the early stages of Alzheimer's disease, out on a limb. The worker, sensing that Margaret is disconnecting from the group, provides her and all the other members the opportunity to react. When Sarah tries to explain the advice she gave, it only heightens Margaret's sense that she has nothing important to say and does not belong in the group. The worker then turns to the group and asks for feedback.

CONCLUSION AND IMPLICATIONS

The number of family caregivers will continue growing dramatically for the foreseeable future. Programs designed to support them are opening throughout the country and outside of the United States. Caregiver support groups are often included as one of the services offered. While most caregivers do not attend a group, a significant number do participate. That number should grow as younger people, who are more familiar with the concept of support groups, become caregivers. This situation provides great opportunity for group work. Caregiver concerns and issues fit beautifully into the scope and purpose of support groups.

To get the most out of a group, caregivers must be able to rely on workers who are knowledgeable about both group work and caregiver problems, themes and issues. The skilled worker will help members who might have very different backgrounds and experiences find common ground despite significant differences. This will not be done by smoothing over conflicts but by encouraging open discussion and exploration of differing opinions and experiences. Workers who incorporate into their practice Northen and Kurland's essential beliefs on the value of differences in a group will succeed in helping the group benefit all members. Also essential is information about the issues that will arise in a caregiver support group. A thorough understanding of the emotions and feelings underpinning many of the issues and familiarity with community resources and entitlements will be most helpful.

Since many caregiver support groups go on for years and see new members join and old members leave, more exploration is needed on this type of group. How do group stages evolve and what special skills are needed for workers facilitating such a group? Also important is comparing groups which are more homogenous to those with more diverse membership. For example, there are support groups for husbands, for people caring for a relative in a nursing home or for wives caring for a husband with dementia. Other groups accept all caregivers. What are the strengths and weaknesses of both types of support groups? Caregivers and programs for them are here to stay. Group workers with skills and knowledge are needed to work with support groups that help sustain caregivers throughout their caregiving career.

REFERENCES

Bertcher, H.J. and Maple, F. (1985). Elements and issues in group composition. In Sundel, M., Glasser, P., Sarri, R. and Vinter, R. (Eds.), *Individual change through small groups* (pp. 180-202). New York: The Free Press.

Feder, J., Komisar, H.L. and Niefeld, M. (2000). Long-term care in the United States: An overview. *Health Affairs*, 19 (3), 40-56.

Fredman, L. and Daly, M.P. (1998). Enhancing practitioner ability to recognize and treat caregiver physical and mental consequences. *Topics in Geriatric Rehabilitation*, 14 (1), 36-44.

Gearing, R.E. (2002). Gender diversity: A powerful tool for enriching group experience. In Henry, S., East, J. and Schmitz, C. (Eds.) *Social work with groups: Mining the gold* (pp. 89-104). Binghamton New York: The Haworth Press, Inc.

Henry J. Kaiser Family Foundation, Harvard School of Public Health, United Hospital Fund of New York and Visiting Nurse Service of New York (2002, June). *The wide circle of caregiving, key findings from a national survey: Long-term care from the caregiver's perspective.* Author.

Houts, P.S., Nezu, A.M., Nezu, C.M. and Bucher, J.A. (1996). The prepared family caregiver: A problem-solving approach to family caregiver education. *Patient Education and Counseling*, 27, 63-73.

Kelly, T.B. and Berman-Rossi, T. (1999). Advancing stages of group development theory: The care of institutionalized older persons. *Social Work with Groups*, 22(2/3), 119-138.

Kurland, R. and Salmon, R. (1997). When worker and member expectations collide: The dilemma of establishing group norms in conflicted situations. In Alissi, A.S., Corto Mergins, C.G. (Eds.) *Voices from the field: Group work responds* (pp. 43-53) Binghamton, NY: The Haworth Press, Inc.

Kurland, R. and Salmon, R. (1998). *Teaching a methods course in social work with groups.* Alexandria, VA: CSWE.

McCallion, P. and Toseland, R.W. (1995). Supportive group interventions with caregivers of frail older adults. In Galinsky, M. J. and Schopler, J.H. (Eds.), *Support groups: Current perspectives on theory and practice* (pp. 11-25). Binghamton, NY: The Haworth Press, Inc.

Mui, A. C. and Burnette, D.J. (1994). A comparative profile of frail elderly persons living alone and those living with others. *Journal of Gerontological Social Work*, 21 (3/4), 5-26.

Northen, H. and Kurland, R. (2001). *Social work with groups* (Third edition). New York: Columbia University Press.

Polivka, L. (2005). The ethics and politics of caregiving. *The Gerontologist*, 45 (4), 557-561.

Satow, R. (2005). *Doing the right thing: Taking care of your elderly parents even if they didn't take care of you.* New York: Jeremy P. Tarcher/Penguin.

Schopler, J.H. and Galinsky, M.J. (1995). Expanding our view of support groups as open systems. In Galinsky, M. J. and Schopler, J.H. (Eds.), *Support groups: Current perspectives on theory and practice* (pp. 3-10). Binghamton, NY: The Haworth Press, Inc.

Schulz, R., O'Brien, A.T., Bookwala, J. and Fleissner, K., (1995). Psychiatric and physical morbidity effects of dementia caregiving: Prevalence, correlates, and causes. *The Gerontologist*, 35, 771-791.

Steinberg, D. M. (2004). *The mutual-aid approach to working with groups: Helping people help each other* (Second edition). Binghamton, New York: The Haworth Press, Inc.

Toseland, R.W. (1995). *Group work with the elderly and family caregivers.* New York: Springer Publishing Company, Inc.

Group Bereavement Support for Spouses Who Are Grieving the Loss of a Partner to Cancer

Rachel M. Schneider

SUMMARY. This paper describes how a time-limited, closed bereavement support group for spouses and significant others was developed at a large, urban cancer center that had not had any formalized bereavement program for some time. This group was created in an attempt to reach out to people who were experiencing the appropriately difficult responses to grief after the loss of a loved one. This paper presents lessons and "best practices" derived from this experience, suggests standards for pre-group planning, and offers a glimpse of how a bereavement group can be especially beneficial to spouses within the first year of loss. *[Article copies available for a fee from The Haworth Document Delivery Service: 1-800-HAWORTH. E-mail address: <docdelivery@haworthpress.com> Website: <http://www.HaworthPress.com> © 2006 by The Haworth Press, Inc. All rights reserved.]*

KEYWORDS. Bereavement, spousal support group, group work in oncology setting, mutual-aid, pre-group planning, time-limited group, beginnings, middles, endings

---

[Haworth co-indexing entry note]: "Group Bereavement Support for Spouses Who Are Grieving the Loss of a Partner to Cancer." Schneider, Rachel M. Co-published simultaneously in *Social Work with Groups* (The Haworth Press, Inc.) Vol. 29, No. 2/3, 2006, pp. 259-278; and: *Making Joyful Noise: The Art, Science, and Soul of Group Work* (ed: Andrew Malekoff, Robert Salmon, and Dominique Moyse Steinberg) The Haworth Press, Inc., 2006, pp. 259-278. Single or multiple copies of this article are available for a fee from The Haworth Document Delivery Service [1-800-HAWORTH, 9:00 a.m. - 5:00 p.m. (EST). E-mail address: docdelivery@haworthpress.com].

doi:10.1300/J009v29n02_17

At a comprehensive cancer center, care should not terminate when the life of a patient ends. A patient undergoing cancer treatment and end-of-life care is–understandably–the center of attention for the medical team and for the family caregivers. But when the outcome is death, and the ill person is no longer center stage, what supports–if any–can we as providers offer the surviving spouse and significant others who have been such integral parts of a patient's care team?

In oncology settings, while the cancer patient is being treated, these intimates are typically present for important meetings with physicians and other members of the healthcare team. At this time, spouses and significant others may be offered caregiver support and educational groups to promote their understanding of the disease, improve the quality of the ancillary care they may be giving, and help them cope with their own feelings of distress. Spouses play a crucial role at the interface with hospital staff; they are called upon to make critical healthcare decisions when the patients themselves are incapacitated.

But too often the death of the patient marks the end of the spouse's relationship with the medical team and the cancer center. Most support groups in oncology settings focus on changes that affect the lives of the patient and family during treatment. "Although such programs are effective for meeting the needs of patients and family members while the patient is alive, there are often no available services for family members once the patient has died" (Goldstein et al., 1996, p. 233). Ironically, at this moment of greatest crisis, the support provided to the family abruptly diminishes, sometimes coming to a complete halt. Not only do medical personnel tend to tacitly sever ties with the surviving spouse, but treatment institutions generally neglect to offer necessary bereavement supports because the family is no longer considered part of the "hospital system."

This paper describes how a time-limited, closed bereavement support group for spouses and significant others was developed at a large, urban cancer center that had not had any formalized bereavement program for some time. This group was created in an attempt to reach out to people who were experiencing the appropriately difficult responses to grief after the loss of a loved one. As grieving can affect individuals in various ways, the development of the group was also an opportunity to identify those people who were experiencing more complicated grief.[1]

The cancer center gathered a psychosocial committee made up of members with a special interest in bereavement work. The committee decided that the first spousal support group would be co-led by a clinical social worker and a psychiatrist. This paper presents lessons and "best practices" derived from this experience, suggests standards for pre-group planning, and offers a glimpse of how a bereavement group can be especially beneficial to spouses within the first year of loss.

Families often make enormous changes in their lives in order to provide care to a loved one who is being treated for a life-threatening illness. Individuals often have to make household adjustments, alterations to their work lives and changes in child care, all in an effort to cope with the challenges of supporting a partner whose disease is end stage. It is particularly important that clinical social workers provide this special subset–for simplicity, referred to here as "spouses"–with adequate bereavement services after they have endured the death of a partner.

WHY A GROUP?

Individual psychotherapy and grief counseling are offered to patients' bereaved families with great frequency. Research and clinical experience show that these can be effective treatments in helping people cope with such a significant loss. However, *group support* is a modality of treatment widely thought to be most useful when working with people who are experiencing isolation and loss. Practitioners highlight this notion.

> Group psychotherapy is particularly suited to addressing problems of social isolation and the development of new social networks. Group participants often experience relief through intimate sharing, feeling accepted by a group, realizing that others share their dilemmas, developing new social skills, feelings useful to others, being inspired by others who have found ways of surviving, coping with, and even growing from bereavement. (Lieberman and Yalom, 1989, p. 123)

WHAT KIND OF GROUP IS NEEDED?

Homogeneous. A randomly gathered group is inadequate to serving the needs of this population of grieving spouses. Although there is likely benefit from participation in a heterogeneous support group–that is, one composed of people suffering a range of significant losses–limiting membership to people experiencing similar losses will increase its effectiveness. The literature reinforces a direct relationship between homogeneity and group cohesion in this population. Shared social factors can lead to heightened sharing of personal problems (Hartford, 1971). Homogeneous groups increase the potential for people to relate to one another during intimate discussion and raise members' desire to socialize outside the group based on feelings of commonality. We know that a group of compatible individuals will enjoy higher levels of cohesion and therefore better outcomes. Homogeneous groups offer a basic level of interpersonal compatibility (Yalom, 1995).

Time-limited. Having a short-term group, in this case, for eight consecutive weeks, has several key advantages for the center's population. First, a longer-term group runs the risk of overwhelming potential participants. For some, any long-term commitment to a program at the cancer center can remind them of the many months spent in the hospital during their spouse's treatment. Joining a group which runs over the course of two months is more manageable at a point in a grieving spouse's life when he/she is marking time very carefully. By the same token, grieving individuals are often advised not to make any major life changes or commitments during the first year of loss. A short-term program therefore does not undercut this idea. And, perhaps most importantly, a bereavement group should be a launching point for grief work, rather than a method of resolving the grief entirely. There is no cure for the feelings of loss; there are only instruments to help in navigating the grieving process.

PLANNING AND ASSEMBLING

Kurland and Salmon (1999) emphasize the necessity for pre-group planning and its distinct role as the first real stage of a group's development. In fact, they point out that a lack of careful planning can result in the premature demise of groups. However, as Northen (1988) points out, despite the fact that planning is such a critical component in the design of this modality of treatment, it is very often overlooked by practitioners. Although it is rarely noted, the planning phase also has the benefit of helping to decrease workers' pre-group anxieties. Apart from the needs assessment itself, the planning for the cancer center's bereavement group included three important components: recruitment, individual interviews, and pre-group meetings of the co-therapists.

Recruitment. Although there is a clear need for a bereavement group of this nature at a large cancer center, it can be very difficult to identify spouses who may be interested in participating. There are several key reasons for this.

(1) Medical staff resistance. First and foremost (and often over-looked): medical professionals (and by this I refer to all members of the treatment team) often have difficulty maintaining relationships with the surviving spouses of a deceased patient. Their own difficult feelings about losing a patient after intense treatment can be a barrier to offering surviving family members the support they need. The anxiety of having to face the anger, sadness, despair and disappointment in the surviving loved ones, and perhaps their own personal experiences of loss can cre-ate enormous obstacles to making this necessary contact.

Physicians and nurses are trained to treat and cure illness and disease. The death of a patient can therefore be quite difficult to bear. For this reason, the co-therapists found it especially useful to make frequent and direct contact with the medical teams. The therapists encouraged them to stay alert for recently widowed spouses who met group participation criteria. It was important to educate the staff about the benefits of such a support group and the comfort the doctors and nurses could provide to someone simply by reaching out to offer such bereavement services. In addition, medical staff was aware of the therapists' availability to assist them in ventilating their own difficult and often suppressed feelings pre- and post-contact with grieving spouses.

(2) Advertising the group was a particularly difficult task. Given the center's mission to advance the research and cure of cancer, the culture of the hospital does not support large public advertisements of death and be-reavement. I was also concerned about the effect that public flyers or other displays could have on other patients and families who were under-going active cancer treatments. Ultimately, we designed a card which de-scribed all available bereavement programs, including individual and group support and provided necessary contact information. As the social workers routinely send cards to families after the death of a loved one, we asked that they included the new insert as well.

We provided only general guidelines to faculty who would be part of our recruitment effort in order to cast our membership net as wide as possible. We asked faculty to consider for the group any person who lost a spouse/partner/significant other after treatment at our institution. We intentionally did not specify an age range or a requirement regard-ing the amount of time since the death in the hopes that this would en-courage staff to refer *any* bereaved spouses who they imagined could benefit from participation in this group.

Pre-group contact. Approximately 12 people expressed initial interest in group participation. All 12 were referrals made by hospital social work staff. One of the co-therapists made telephone contact with each individual to introduce the program, both to provide practical information so they might know what to expect regarding the group structure, content and membership and to develop an initial rapport. Telephone calls typically lasted between 15 and 30 minutes, during which time widows/widowers were encouraged to share some information regarding their loss and the process of grieving. In some cases, people expressed gratitude for the contact and asked for time to process the information/invitation prior to making an appointment to meet for a pre-group interview at the hospital.

Intimacy can develop even during this very first contact. One woman who had lost her female partner six months prior to the telephone call said, "This is such strange timing. I had a dream about Holly last night in which she told me to get myself some help. She said 'I'm here to assist you in doing that.' And, now I get this phone call!" One man who was grieving the death of his wife who passed away eight months earlier said, "I'm pretty surprised to hear from you. I found it pretty disappointing that the hospital hadn't offered me any bereavement programs after Pamela passed away. Is there a reason why this is the first such phone call I'm receiving?" The tension expressed during this conversation represented some members' more negative feelings about the center's response to their intense losses. Discussions such as this one helped to prepare the therapists for negative feedback. They also offered an opportunity for the spouses to overcome disappointment over the lack of services that merely compounded their life-changing loss.

The next step in the pre-group planning process was for the co-therapists to meet together with each potential member in order to hear his or her stories, provide further information about the group and assess the individual's appropriateness for participation. As Lorenz (1998) says, it is important to assess a potential participant's present coping ability, individuals' expectations and reasons for interest at this time, former group experiences, and any special problems such as a psychiatric history or active substance abuse which might make the support group setting inappropriate. Those signing up for participation in the group should have an actual desire to be with other people during this experience and a basic ability to express their thoughts and feelings (Goldstein et al., 1996).

The therapists allotted one hour for every session, during which time each potential member gave an account of the journey he/she took with his/her partner from diagnosis to end of life. People were consistently forthcoming with their personal stories and seemingly open to the possibility of processing these experiences in a group setting. One woman brought a beautiful scrapbook of photographs and writings she had created as a tribute to her female partner, who had been a writer and poet. She walked us through each page, making sure not to leave out any critical aspects of Rose's whole life.

These pre-group sessions were the most critical piece of the planning phase (Hartford, 1971). We were able to spend time with each person in order to develop an understanding of his/her particular loss and the ways in which individuals hoped the group would help them to cope. It is important to note that as the group therapists, we too were initially resistant to holding these individual meetings. We knew that they would be time-consuming (thus taking us away from other work obligations) and potentially emotionally difficult. It was not until the individual meetings were in progress that we recognized their real benefit.

The therapists met after each of these sessions in order to process the experience and make decisions regarding each person's appropriateness for attending the group. We then made telephone contact with each potential member in order to formally invite each one to join the group, and to provide logistics of where and when the first meeting would be held.

People were surprisingly willing to come forward and reach for help in navigating the grieving process during a particularly painful and vulnerable time. Clinical social workers, and others dealing with the terminally ill, are often asked how it remains possible to work so closely with the dying and the bereaved. These pre-group interviews were a wonderful example of how much strength and bravery exists within the human spirit. In the middle of an agonizing journey, these individuals were able to seek connection despite the fact that in many ways a bereavement group subjected them to further vulnerability. Hearing their goals and wishes helped us to develop a firmer sense of how the group could be helpful to members. Equipped with some of their expectations, we were better prepared to create a space that could meet the needs of this particular group.

Co-therapy meetings. Discussion time between co-therapists is an essential ingredient to successful work together (Yalom, 1995). Meeting as co-therapists regularly throughout this process proved useful in helping us to recognize our own countertransferential responses that emerged even during the planning stages. We continued to meet consistently during the group's lifespan in order to process the evolving dynamics and openly discuss our own reactions to the material. We found it optimal to meet briefly just before each group session and then to touch base again at the evening's close. In addition, we were sure to make contact during the days in between meetings as we felt necessary.

Group composition. Of the twelve people who initially showed interest in participating, five did not respond to follow-up phone calls and attempts to meet. Ultimately, seven people confirmed their participation in the group, agreeing to attend all eight sessions. Of the seven, there were five women and two men. As it turned out, all had been legally married, except for two women who had been involved in long-term relationships with a man and woman respectively. All had lost their spouses between two and twelve-months prior to the group's beginning. Only two members had had any prior group participation experience. One woman joined a community-based spousal support group while she was also participating in this group.

As facilitators we made members aware of our ongoing availability should they have any concerns as the group sessions got underway. We explained the benefits of attending all eight sessions and asked that members contact us should they feel that the group in any way was not meeting their needs. We also asked if any one considered terminating prematurely, at any point, that they process their feelings with us so that we could attempt to meet their needs and/or assist them in achieving a higher degree of comfort in the group. As it turned out, no one openly contemplated early termination.

ESTABLISHING A THERAPEUTIC TONE/IDENTITY FOR THE GROUP

Because most of the group members had never attended a support group, and certainly none had attended a bereavement support group, it was important to assist them in acclimating right from the start. It is critical to the leader's role to attempt to mitigate initial anxiety by helping members to see their role within the context of the group (Lorenz, 1998). In this milieu it was especially important to create an environment that would help people to achieve an optimal comfort level in the room. This included making explicit basic expectations such as maintaining the group's confidentiality and respecting other people's grieving process and rituals.

We decided to hold group meetings in an administrative building across the street from the main hospital that houses inpatient units and outpatient clinics. The rationale behind this was straightforward; we wanted to decrease the potential for the re-traumatization that could occur were we to bring people back to the very place where their dead spouses were treated. In addition, we hoped that even the small geographic separation from the hospital would give members permission to openly share any negative feelings toward the center and/or medical staff.

We made it clear, too, that in contradistinction from other groups they might have participated in or heard about, we *encouraged* outside contact among members. Many groups have strict regulations about this, but we explained that it was up to them to make that decision for themselves. Taking it a step further, and with the idea in mind that this group could help to decrease people's social isolation, we provided examples of ways in which people might want to have social interactions with one another. We felt it important to convey our understanding that people might want to have further contact with one another outside of the hour-and-a half group sessions (Caserta and Lund, 1996).

THE WORK OF THE GROUP

From the very first session, the group started working to confront painful issues and speak openly about a variety of difficult topics. Among these were themes that the group continued to work on intensely together throughout the eight-week period. These included: personal rationale for participation, issues related to group termination, conflicted feelings about looking toward the future, change in social roles, and methods of coping with the severity of painful feelings.

Why am I here? In the first session, we asked each member to share as much as he or she wanted to about the loss, what drew him or her to participate in a spousal bereavement support group and what each hoped to get out of the experience. Participants described in some detail the history of their partners' illnesses and the specific circumstances surrounding the death. When several members, understandably, became tearful while disclosing this difficult material, others were quick to pass around tissues or offer a gesture of understanding. Each person listened carefully to everyone else's accounts, and either verbally or through body language conveyed a sense of compassion and provided the comfort of mutual aid. Knowing that the experiences of grief are shared by other group members can make the associated feelings somewhat less frightening and therefore easier to confront in the room (Shulman, 1992).

Members tended to echo each other's sentiments about the desire to attend a support group of this type. "I feel like I'm burning out my friends. I'm sure they don't want to listen over and over again to all of my problems; to how sad I am," one man said. This comment was met with resounding words of understanding. This was a fear to which all members could strongly relate. Another woman said, "As much as people try to be supportive–and believe me they do, they really do–they can't possibly know what it is that I'm going through. I guess that's what I'm hoping to find here–a small community of people who just know and really get what this is really like."

By and large, everyone expressed a strong need to be in the presence of other people who had the capacity for truly understanding their first-hand grief. Several members stated they hoped that the group would be a space where they could share their thoughts about grieving without fear of being judged. One woman said that she saw this group as an opportunity to expand her social circle in a meaningful way, that it could help decrease the overwhelming sense of loneliness she has felt since her spouse died. She reported that the isolation she experienced with the loss of her partner was so great that she had an urgent need to simply feel connected to other human beings again.

Another woman openly displayed her ambivalence about attending a support program at all. Five months earlier she had lost her husband of fifteen years and stated that she'd had "major reservations" about participating in this group, but her psychotherapist encouraged her to "give it a try." She felt cautious that hearing other members' tales of loss could leave her feeling re-traumatized at a critical time in her own healing. Another member concurred; he too worried about feeling "worse after leaving the group" as a result of bearing witness to other people's pain. It is noteworthy that, by the second session, many members described feeling *better* than they had anticipated feeling after the first night. They reported a sense of surprise with the comfort and sense of belonging that they experienced.

Levy and Derby (1992) state that it is common for some bereaved individuals to fear this sort of involvement because they think their own grief will only be exacerbated when they are exposed to other people's painful stories. One woman who was widowed after thirty years of "a wonderful marriage" revealed that she was finally ready to hear other people's tales of loss, and believed that she could now help others confront their own complicated emotions. She added that in spite of her own grief, she has developed methods of coping with uncomfortable feelings and wants to share these skills with others. Casting herself in the role of mentor felt to her like a therapeutic opportunity.

Termination. Beginning stages of any group are typically fraught with ambivalence even in the best of circumstances. At this phase, members usually have a desire for closeness, but are fearful of it as well. Individuals' anxiety about their own acceptance and vulnerability tends to be quite high. It is, therefore, a time when people actively question how much they can trust the group (Kurland and Salmon, 1999). The example of the group member whose psychotherapist urged her to attend illustrates this point well. Prior to the initial group meeting, she was questioning the appropriateness of her attendance and was already starting to ask herself (and her therapist) whether she would actually gain anything from participating. The fact that she openly expressed this initial apprehension to the group during so early on speaks to the level of ambivalence she was experiencing.

With careful listening a therapist can usually hear issues of termination arise at this early stage. However, when the purpose of the group itself is to assist people in coping with the end of a primary relationship, issues of group termination are, not surprisingly, particularly palpable. Termination, rather than presenting itself as a distinct stage in the group's development, and one that tends to emerge in ending stages of a group, was an ongoing theme which crept into the very first session and was discussed in nearly every session up to the last group meeting. During the termination phase, members tend to demonstrate their fears of losing the group, the progress made and perhaps even the support of the therapists. In non-bereavement groups, the termination phase is typically marked by members identifying more satisfying outside relationships, thus causing them to loosen ties with the group itself. In contrast, with grieving individuals, members are in the group because they are mourning the loss of their most important relationship and are therefore are likely more ambivalent about the loss of the group itself (Kurland and Salmon, 1999).

One particularly articulate and vocal group member asked us directly about our decision to keep the group to eight 1.5 hour sessions. He spoke openly about the extraordinary pain of losing a spouse after cancer treatment and stated clearly that eight weeks felt *"like a tease,"* and certainly *"an insufficient amount of time to appropriately move through the grieving process."* His tone was a combination of disappointment and rage. While we listened carefully to his concerns about a time-limited bereavement group, we also made explicit the reasons for keeping to the frame. We used this as an opportunity to deepen the work by trying to gain a fuller understanding of what the short-term approach meant to him and to the other group members.

As group therapists, we were prepared to listen closely to what was not being said as a means of hearing any early feelings related to the process of termination. We were relieved that despite the fact that in this beginning phase members were struggling to develop their own voices in the room, they were nonetheless comfortable enough to articulate negative feelings about the group's inevitable end.

> Members react to this stage with anger, denial, regression, and flight. Attendance can fall off as members start to disengage; criticisms of the group, the leader, or other members may be expressed; members can be clingy, asking why the group has to end, or may become detached and removed. (Goelitz, 2004, pp. 213-214)

As the discussion of ending arose at the group's beginning, it was particularly important to pay close attention to signs of potential disengagement and flight. Fortunately, members were able to work through the complexities of this issue energetically without threatening to leave. Instead, they each expressed feelings about wanting the group to continue for a longer period of time. Interestingly, despite the fact that at this point they did not yet know how they would ultimately feel about the group, they were already advocating for its being lengthened. This underscored members' general sense of anxiety in attaching to a new set of people and developing new relationships. Holland (2000, p. 294) states, "Grief is the price of those attachments of love that we make in our lives."

In that first session, people wanted to learn more about the decision to keep the length of the group to eight weeks and if we, as facilitators, felt that they would be at a particular point in their grieving by the time it needed to end. Members expressed their ambivalence about participating in something that had a certain endpoint, and wanted assurance that they would be "healed" or that their grief would be "fixed" by the time the group ended. Not only was it impossible to make such a promise to them, but we also emphasized that this sort of loss takes a long time to mourn.

For facilitators, managing issues of termination so early on in a group's development can be very difficult. Goelitz (2004) discusses leaders' own reactions to termination and the unconscious efforts often made to prolong the group. During the fourth meeting of this bereavement group, we demonstrated our own feelings of ambivalence by openly considering extending the group timeframe by two to three weeks. The idea emerged from ongoing group discussions, and, because of our own responses we nearly missed the opportunity to reach for deeper feelings about it rather than attempting to find a cure for the problem. We allowed a debate to ensue. Thus, we revealed our own ambivalence regarding the group's inevitable end. Moreover, by displaying our own ambivalence, we allowed people to hold out hope for a less difficult conclusion. This only made more difficult the group's struggle with the feelings associated with endings and the sense of loss that they anticipated feeling.

As in the planning stages, we continued to spend time before and after each session processing the group content together. In so doing, we were able to tease out our own discomfort with the issue of termination and recognized that we were trying to protect members (and ourselves) from being traumatized by yet another loss. Ultimately, we made our own feelings explicit to the group and made it clear that we would have to stick to the original eight-week timeline. By the fifth group meeting, as participants expressed their frustration with us, and with the circumstances, we feared that the group might simply disintegrate. To our surprise, participants appeared to have reached a higher level of cohesion and demonstrated an enormous amount of flexibility and resilience in their ability to manage the chaos associated with this conflicted discussion.

By these middle sessions, people were sharing personal feelings at a high rate, displaying a tremendous amount of trust and intimacy. The meetings were energized, and both members and workers noted that "the time seemed to fly." Members consistently asked each other about family members and outside activities by name, thus demonstrating both a level of comfort and a genuine interest in the others' outside lives. At this point in the group's lifespan we began laughing together too. People shared funny stories of present day significance and sometimes also looked back and recounted earlier experiences with their spouses. The focus, we had predicted and hoped, shifted from recounting the circumstances of early grief and managing the shock and agony of loss to looking ahead and thinking about what they hoped for themselves in the future.

LOOKING TOWARDS THE FUTURE

One woman who was particularly introverted and always more reserved than the others was surprisingly the one to broach a particularly taboo subject. She asked the other members how they felt about the possibility of dating other people. "I don't mean right now," she was quick to assert, "I just mean in general . . . at some point." There was visible relief in the room once this question was asked. It was clear that although everyone had contemplated this privately, none had thus far been able to raise the topic in the room. Bereaved spouses often fear that making significant changes and developing new relationships could make them feel as though they are betraying their dead partner (Lieberman and Yalom, 1989). People often feel guilty that they are able to enjoy any interpersonal interactions or social events.

Once the topic of new relationships was firmly on the table, one woman admitted that she had begun to spend time with a man she had met while away for a weekend retreat. She assured the group that she had not had any physical involvement with him thus far, however, but had begun to "really enjoy his company." It quickly became clear that even "casual" involvement with another potential partner made her worry that she was betraying her late spouse.

Another woman stated that she had begun to look at men on the crosstown bus and contemplate which characteristics she felt most drawn to. She was surprised to realize that she had not dated, or even thought about dating, since she was a young adult, and she expressed feeling scared at the prospect embarking into the world of single people. She also voiced feelings of guilt regarding her own ability to "forget" about her husband during the few minutes she spent looking at other men. However, she was quick to add that she knew she had been through very difficult times, felt proud about the care she had provided her husband while he was ill and felt strongly that she should not have to suffer for the rest of her life as a result of having lost him so early in their lives together. Other group members assured her that she was entitled to feel pleasure again. Moreover, they actively supported "her right" to reclaim happiness in her life. The taboo nature of this topic was mitigated as the group worked together to explore deeper and perhaps more difficult feelings (Shulman, 1992).

As comfort with this topic began to increase, so too did the level of participation in the discussion. The group began openly sharing feelings about dating and developing romantic feelings toward new potential love interests. During the course of the eight weeks, none had begun a new romantic relationship, yet each revealed feelings about exploring that territory at some point in the future. The safety of the group environment allowed individuals to take the risk of considering this idea "publicly." Several widows/widowers stated that prior to speaking openly in this room about the possibility of developing new relationships; they had experienced an increased sense of guilt and anxiety as a result of even harboring such thoughts. Once made explicit in the group context, they were able to contemplate the mixture of feelings associated with their desire for a future intimate relationship. Group members helped each other to accept the complicated feelings but also to acknowledge the positive aspects of desiring a future intimate relationship.

ROLE SHIFTS

> The death of a spouse has long been recognized as one of the most stressful life experiences in the intensity and duration of the mourning process and in the required readjustments to life roles. (Marmar et al., 1997, p. 203)

The theme of role shifts emerged continually in the group room. Each participant had been intimately involved in his/her partner's care during illness and then the end of life. Most members described having been cast into the role of caretaker or nurse and thus having given up aspects of their earlier roles as spouse, partner, lover, and friend. When their spouses died, each faced yet another new and distinct role, that of widow or widower. The group examined the feelings associated with the loss of the "we," the loss of being a part of a couple.

A man whose adult children are living with him at home asked the group how others were dealing with being in their houses without their spouses. Group members poured forth conflicted feelings. Some people expressed fear of being home alone at night or during particularly difficult days. One widow quietly said that she felt some relief that there was no longer a hospital bed and medical equipment in the home; that she felt peaceful at night when she was by herself. One woman said that she hadn't thought much yet about her actual home and said that a more difficult thing for her has been having to reach out to single friends to avoid feeling "like a fifth wheel when out with other couples." Other members were quick to add that this new state of aloneness meant having to consider their own needs and desires after years of taking care of someone else. The group itself served as a launching pad for people to begin identifying their own wishes and goals for the future. As the group demonstrated an interest in one individual's feelings, each participant began to recognize and then articulate some of his or her unique, individual desires.

This shift represented an important and difficult adjustment for group members. For some it meant the painful confrontation of life without a mate; for others it meant admitting out loud that they felt a sense of freedom at being able to explore their individuality and singleness. One woman stated that she had gotten so used to scheduling her days around her husband's needs as he became increasingly incapacitated that she actively missed having someone to care for; to look after. She stated that she did not want to address her own needs; that her own needs consisted of taking care of her husband.

Perhaps one of the most difficult things for the group to confront was the sense that they were each able to do certain things that they could not do before. For all, the burden of caring for a partner over a long-term illness meant giving up some or all of their own needs. For some, however, the illness was not the first time that they put their own desires on hold. One man confessed that even when his wife was well, she was less social than he, which often propelled him to give up activities he had enjoyed in his life prior to marriage. One woman spoke with pride about all her new "firsts" (the first time she slept alone in their vacation home, the first time she asked a friend out to a concert). She had never been on her own before, and although she missed her husband dearly she was finding pleasure in discovering some of her own hidden skills and talents. She watched herself take risks she had never before imagined taking.

Members were grappling with their shifting roles in different ways. One man described his need to reprioritize his work life now that he was the sole caretaker of a ten-year-old child. "Before taking leave to care for my wife, I never thought twice about accepting work assignments that kept me traveling for several days at a clip. Now I have Jenny to consider, and couldn't possibly imagine being away from her for that long. I'm going to have to insist on only taking projects that are local, so that I can be home in time to make dinner."

One widow said that she was going to need to learn to drive, which was something she always put off and was afraid to do. "I guess the time has come! I'm going to have to take a deep breath and give it a try." In both of these cases, and in many others, people were confronting the need to make changes in their lives that would shift their own self-image.

COPING WITH DIFFICULT FEELINGS

Tolerating intensely painful feelings of loss and sadness was something that the group faced during each meeting. It took a great deal of strength as individuals and as a unit to confront this together. Many began talking about their frustrations with not being able to speed up the grieving process. For example, a 42-year-old widower asked directly for information on how long one should continue to grieve, how much time one should spend focusing on a deceased spouse, how soon one could consider returning to work or to other areas of life that had been "put on hold." In essence, he was asking for a prescription for how long and how deeply one should be entrenched in the process of grieving and wanted permission to think about the next phase of his life.

It was our responsibility as facilitators to provide the group with information about the process of grief, which tends not to follow one particular pattern. As the therapists, we thought it was important to emphasize that the grieving process necessarily takes time and that it is not advisable to try and speed it up (Lorenz, 1998). By the same token, we provided a description of more complicated grieving patterns so that members could be aware of what to look out for and when to consider seeking further assistance in coping with their losses. For the most part, however, group members expressed an understanding and insight into the notion that there is no "right path" to follow. By asking facilitators for the answers or a magic pill as one member joked, they were highlighting the difficulty they had in not having one map to follow. The encouragement we were able to offer, however, was that in contrast to the trajectory for a psychiatric illness, grief experienced after the loss of a spouse will show marked improvement over time (Lieberman and Yalom, 1989).

CONCLUSION

"Bereavement support is an essential element in the provision of comprehensive oncology care" (Lorenz, 1998, p. 165). Unfortunately, it is also one of the areas most often overlooked in cancer centers and those providing services to oncology patients and their families. This paper describes why it is important and worthwhile to confront the inevitable institutional hurdles in order to meet the needs of bereaved spouses. The resistance to creating bereavement groups such as the one described here remains high, especially at institutions whose mission is to advance the treatment of cancer patients. The reality is that as baby boomers age, cancer becomes more prevalent in our population. And, unfortunately, despite the fact that new treatment options are emerging all the time, people will continue to lose loved ones after difficult battles with the disease. Oncology settings therefore will continue to have an obligation to provide solid bereavement services to family members.

As our experience makes clear, it is only through pre-group conceptualizing and planning that a successful group can develop. We learned that pre-contact via telephone and in person was instrumental in developing a sense of belonging trust early on in the group's lifespan. Although these components are often seen as highly time-consuming and can be taxing on workers, they are necessary to a group's successful development. As an ancillary benefit, participating in the process of pre-group planning decreases anxiety for group workers and new bereavement workers.

By the last session of the group, members expressed sadness about ending and some anxiety about what the next steps might be for them in their grief processes. Despite these difficult feelings, they openly thanked one another for listening and for helping them to cope with their painful losses. In addition, they thanked one another for sharing so openly their personal stories and complicated emotions.

At this last session, each member completed a multiple-choice survey, a tool we used in an effort to collect information about how to enhance the program for future groups. By and large, the group members expressed positive feelings about having participated and stated that they planned to attempt to stay in touch and connect with one another outside of the group. Some members commented that they were struck by the lack of conflict in the room. As leaders, we were unsure whether the lack of conflict was a result of being polite with one another or because their small, personal gripes with one another were subordinate to the greater purpose of being present.

The member who had raised the issue of termination in the very first session laughed and said, "You know you'll get no argument from me! I'm the person who has been fighting for more time together since the beginning!"

NOTE

1. An extremely close or conflictual relationship with the deceased may lead to complicated or unresolved grief that can be manifest as an inability to experience normal grief reactions (i.e., an absence of grief and mourning), conflicted grief, delayed grief, or chronic grief. An example of complicated grief is when death comes suddenly as in a traumatic event. Normal grief responses of longing for a loved one are then intermingled with alarming memories of the event and may disrupt the usual grief process (Webb, 2004).

REFERENCES

Caserta., M. and Lund, D. (1996). Beyond bereavement support group meetings: Exploring outside social contacts among the members. *Death Studies*, 20(6), 537-556.

Classen, C., Diamond, S., Soleman, A., Fobair, P., Spira, J. and Spiegel, D. (1993). *Brief supportive-expressive group therapy for women with primary breast cancer: A treatment manual*. California: Stanford University School of Medicine.

Ettin, M. (2000). From identified patient to identifiable group: The alchemy of the group as a whole. *International Journal of Group Psychotherapy*, 50(2), 137-162.

Folken, M. (1990). Moderating grief of widowed people in talk groups. *Death Studies*, 14, 171-176.

Goelitz, A. (2004). Using the end of groups as an intervention at end-of-life. *Journal of Gerontological Social Work*, 44(1/2), 211-221.

Goldstein, J. Alter, C. and Axelrod, R. (1996). A psychoeducational bereavement-support group for families provided in an outpatient cancer center. *Journal of Cancer Education*, 11(4), 233-237.

Hartford, M. (1971). *Groups in social work*. New York: Columbia University Press.

Holland, J. and Lewis, S. (2001). *The human side of cancer*. New York: HarperCollins.

Kissane, D. (2004). Bereavement, in Doyle, D., Hanks, G., Cherny, N. and Claman, K. (Eds). *Oxford textbook of palliative medicine, 3rd Ed*. Oxford, UK: Oxford University Press.

Kurland, R. and Salmon, R. (1999). *Teaching a methods course in social work with groups*. Alexandria, VA: Council on Social Work Education

Lawrence, L. (1992). 'Till death do us part': The application of object relations theory to facilitate mourning in a young widows' group. *Social Work in Health Care*, 16(3), 67-81.

Levy, L. and Derby, J. (1992). Bereavement support groups: Who joins; who does not; and why. *American Journal of Community Psychology*, 20(5), 649-662.

Lieberman, M. (1989). Group properties and outcomes: A study of group norms in self-help groups for widows and widowers. *International Journal Group Psychotherapy*, 39(2), 191-208.

Lieberman, M. and Yalom, I. (1992). Brief group psychotherapy for the spousally bereaved: A controlled study. *International Journal of Group Psychotherapy*, 42(1), 117-132.

Lorenz, L. (1998). Selecting and implementing support groups for bereaved adults. *Cancer Practice*, 6(3), 161-166

Marbar, C., Horowitz, M., Weiss, D., Wilner, N. and Kaltreider., N. (1987). Presented at the 140th annual meeting of the American Psychiatric Association, Chicago May 9-14, 1987. Copyright 1988 American Psychiatric Association.

Middleman, R. and Wood, G. (1990). *Skills for direct practice in social work*. New York: Columbia University Press.

Northen, H. (1988). *Social work with groups*. New York: Columbia University Press.

Piper, W., Ogrodniczuk, J., Joyce, A., McCalum, M. and Rosie, J. (2002). Relationships among affect, work, and outcome in group therapy for patients with complicated grief. *American Journal of Psychotherapy*, 56(3), 347-361.

Potocky, M. (1993). Effective services for bereaved spouses. *Health and Social Work*, 18(4), 288-301.

Rose, S. (1989). Coping skill training in groups. *International Journal of Group Psychotherapy*, 39(1), 59-78.

Shulman, L. (1992). *The skills of helping: Individuals, families and groups, 3rd Edition*. Illinois: F.E. Peacock Publishers

Sonnebelt-Smeenge, S. and DeVries, R. (2003). The effects of gender and age on grief work associated with grief support groups. *Illness, Crisis & Loss*, 11(3), 226-241.

Walls, N. and Meyers, A. (1985). Outcome in group treatments for bereavement: Experimental results and recommendations for clinical practice. *International Journal of Mental Health*, 13(3-4), 126-147.

Webb, N. B. (2004). The impact of traumatic stress and loss on children and families. In N. Boyd Webb (Ed). *Mass trauma and violence: Helping families and children cope*. New York: Guilford Press, 3-22.

Yalom, I. (1995). *The theory and practice of group psychotherapy, Fourth Edition*. New York: BasicBooks.

Yalom, I. and Vinogradov, S. (1988). Bereavement groups: Techniques and themes. *International Journal of Group Psychotherapy*, 38(4) 419-446.

Retrospective Book Review:
Teaching a Methods Course in Social Work with Groups

Mary C. Bitel

SUMMARY. Eight years after its publication, *Teaching a Methods Course in Social Work with Groups* serves as a reminder to social workers of group work's historic roots and its value as a method of practice with diverse populations. The author shares her experiences in utilizing the teaching text in her work with MSW students and students of the arts who facilitate activity-based groups in community settings. Citing examples of students' experiences in group work facilitation, the author touches on the constraints emerging group workers face in translating social work skills and values to practice. The author's retrospective review of the teaching text underscores its continued importance in the field of social group work instruction. *[Article copies available for a fee from The Haworth Document Delivery Service: 1-800-HAWORTH. E-mail address: <docdelivery@haworthpress.com> Website: <http://www.HaworthPress.com> © 2006 by The Haworth Press, Inc. All rights reserved.]*

KEYWORDS. Social group work education, group work history, group work skills and values, mutual aid, group work curriculum

---

[Haworth co-indexing entry note]: "Retrospective Book Review: *Teaching a Methods Course in Social Work with Groups*." Bitel, Mary C. Co-published simultaneously in *Social Work with Groups* (The Haworth Press, Inc.) Vol. 29, No. 2/3, 2006, pp. 279-286; and: *Making Joyful Noise: The Art, Science, and Soul of Group Work* (ed: Andrew Malekoff, Robert Salmon, and Dominique Moyse Steinberg) The Haworth Press, Inc., 2006, pp. 279-286. Single or multiple copies of this article are available for a fee from The Haworth Document Delivery Service [1-800-HAWORTH, 9:00 a.m. - 5:00 p.m. (EST). E-mail address: docdelivery@ haworthpress.com].

Upon its publication eight years ago, Carol Cohen (1998) wrote a clear and comprehensive review of *Teaching a Methods Course in Social Work with Groups* for the journal *Social Work with Groups*. Ms. Cohen began her review with the observation that group work was experiencing a state of neglect in schools of social work. She offered that group work practice was increasingly in demand, yet educators lacked advanced knowledge and experience with the specific skills, concepts, and values of social work with groups. Eight years later, groups are increasingly utilized as a method for working with individuals in a wide range of practice settings. In addition to lack of in-depth group work training in schools of social work, new and greater challenges to the health and growth of social group work as a practice modality have gained prominence since the book's publication. Questions regarding its efficacy, expediency, and cost-effectiveness in contemporary practice settings continue to push group work into a model of practice that seldom resembles its settlement house origins as a means for social action, access to the democratic process, and catalyst for individual growth and social connection. Eight years later, *Teaching a Methods Course* serves as a reminder to social workers of group work's historic roots and its value as a method of practice with diverse populations. The text remains vitally important for strengthening and enriching the fields of social group work education and practice.

The value and power of working with groups resonates through *Teaching a Methods Course*. Master's level students who were lucky enough to study with Roselle Kurland and Robert Salmon directly can hear their voices in each unit of the text. Those of us who have gone on to teach group work in a variety of academic and organizational contexts use the authors' words and ideas in every class or training session that we teach. We hear their voices through the case examples offered in each chapter. We hear them in the straightforward approach to teaching group work through stages of group development. We hear them in the discussions on casework in a group; a concept we all struggled with as students and one which continues to challenge us as practitioners and teachers. We use their words to help our own students engage in the struggle to understand the difference between casework in the group and honest-to-goodness group work. But we are the lucky ones. We learned directly from them why it is so important to study the skills and theories of social work with groups before we call ourselves group workers, for as they instructed us and we in turn teach our own students, to do less diminishes the craft, allows for shoddy group work, and does not fully serve those with whom we work in the group setting.

The first time I stepped into a classroom to teach group work the only thing that kept me from walking straight back out the door was the knowledge that I had Kurland and Salmon's teaching book tucked into my briefcase. The authors offer a text that takes the instructor through a one-semester overview of what they suggest to be the "knowledge, values, and skills most crucial to beginning practice in social work with groups." Given the authors' intentions with the book, I knew that I had a mission as an instructor to help infuse MSW students with the joy of facilitating groups. In order to do that, I had to offer them in ten short class sessions the fundamentals of social work with groups and introduce them to the power of groups as a tool for individual and group growth. The *Teaching* text proved extremely valuable in focusing that process. The text provides a straightforward guide for teaching group work that parallels the actual stages of group development. The book flows in such an organic yet carefully structured way that it supports the group work instructor from start to finish and yet provides the space for innovation, use of self, and flexibility in instruction. Beginning with a guide on how to launch a course in group work, through a brief history of group work in the United States, and on through stages of group development, the text is concise yet thorough and so will not scare off the novice instructor. The book is particularly helpful to beginning instructors and fledgling group workers on the subject of pre-group planning and formation, a stage of group work often under-used, under-valued, and misunderstood by practitioners and administrators in professional practice. The book's thorough orientation to this first stage of group development lays the foundation for the concepts that follow. The appendices at the conclusion of the text enhance the core eleven units of instruction and are useful tools for direct application with students.

As Ms. Cohen suggests in her review, the *Teaching* text can provide valuable support to seasoned social work instructors as well. The book never seems to "talk down" to the reader or offer group work pronouncements from on high, but instead takes the group instructor by the elbow and offers encouragement and support for what they might either instinctually know or have learned in MSW level group work instruction. The real gift of this book for group work educators is how it balances between sharing information with new group work instructors and providing a concise primer for more seasoned instructors, with equal respect for both along the teaching continuum.

In my first semester as a group work instructor I used *Teaching a Methods Course* like a Michelin guide to the best spots on a grand tour of group work. I found myself reading the book at every available opportunity, which included my weekly trips uptown on the Number 6 subway line to teach at Hunter College School of Social Work; no small teaching feat as I was following in the footsteps of the two group workers who had literally written the book on how to teach group work . . . and on their own turf, no less. As tourists around me perused their guide books on the highlights of New York City, I would pull out my own guide and thumb through the section on "Dealing with Conflict and Difference," making notes in the margin about my own experiences as a practitioner on that subject. As I became a more seasoned teacher I discovered for myself what Carol Cohen has noted in her original review, that the book could "serve as a cushion" for new instructors to navigate their way over the "personal 'rough spots' with teaching social work practice with groups." Cohen suggests that with each passing experience the group work instructor begins to "be more selective and develop more individual teaching materials" while continuing to use the book as a guide to course organization and progression. I learned in that first semester of teaching, and continue to learn, exactly what I did not know about group work, sometimes in painfully embarrassing ways but always profoundly instructional in nature. But I also learned how to make group work, and the teaching of it, more fully my own. My "rough" spots were cushioned by Kurland and Salmon's enthusiasm for each subject identified in the eleven units that make up the book. Their clear understanding and explication of each skill and concept; their supportive and often humorous suggestions on how to proceed with each subject, and their encouragement to develop an individual approach to teaching the material helped me to balance my own lack of teaching experience with the belief that I had something to offer my students. This is exactly what Salmon and Kurland hoped for with their book. The authors wanted their guide to fuel the instructor's own interest in group work and provide the foundation for the development of a unique teaching style that encompasses the core values, skills, and concepts of social work with groups as provided by them in their text.

About three years ago I developed a course for visual and performing arts students at New York University in response to repeated experiences as an administrator of a community-based after school program for adolescent and teen girls. Our agency welcomed undergraduate and graduate level arts students as interns in various educational and recreational activities that the agency provided in the East Harlem community of New York City. The students possessed all the qualities one could hope for in volunteer staff members: boundless energy, enthusiasm, self-discipline, a desire to learn more about the community in which they volunteered, a sense of social justice, and possibly most important to the program population and setting, a uniquely creative response to group work. What they lacked was an understanding of the specific skills demanded of group workers. As my staff worked with the interns we discovered that those skills were in many ways intuitive; students understood and internalized the value of empathy, the importance of mutual aid, and the necessity for the problem solving process in the group setting. What they needed was a forum for gaining a stronger theoretical grounding in the skills, concepts, and values of social work with groups to match the enthusiasm, creativity, and intuitive connection they already possessed. In a conversation with Roselle Kurland, I shared the idea for a course that would address the skills of social group work with students who were not pursuing a career in social work but held some of the basic values and concepts of social group work in their understanding as artists. Roselle was a hard sell simply for her unfailing dedication to the full and specific teaching of group work and a refusal to compromise her standards for what constituted good group work. Finally, after many conversations, a few futile attempts at a course syllabus, and much muddled thinking, Roselle suggested that I use the *Teaching* book as a ground plan and develop a course that would draw on the important concepts of group work from a uniquely artistic point of view. The *Teaching* book once again became my Michelin guide, but this time to a world that I created out of two equally important parts of my life: the arts and group work. The course utilizes the concepts and skills I have come to understand as the foundation of group work and moves forward to explore purposeful use of activity and the balance of process with task as they impact the visiting artist's work with community groups. Without the authors' equal amounts of unconditional support and demand for me to value the discipline of the craft through my teaching, and *Teaching a Methods Course* as my foundation, I would not have had the tools to pursue something that has become so important to me. It is a truly remarkable and rewarding experience for a former Kurland-Salmon student to be given the opportunity to apply the *Teaching* text to actors, cinematographers, and dancers in a Thursday morning course downtown and apply the very same material to a group of Master's level social work students that same afternoon in a classroom eighty blocks north. It is only after teaching the course for a number of semesters, talking with Roselle Kurland and Robert Salmon about my experiences in teaching both social work students and arts students, and reflecting on their concerns about maintaining the integrity of social group work through instruction and practice that I realize how important those concerns and questions were to the formation of what has become a vitally important part of my professional career as a teacher of group work.

Despite my appreciation of *Teaching a Methods Course*, I do have concerns regarding its contents. Students and colleagues in the field voice concerns regarding the utility of the kind of group work that is supported in the *Teaching* text. The complaint I hear most often is, "This is all well and good, but how can I practice the ideal when I know the reality of the practice landscape?" Group work instructors continue to be challenged to identify group work as a unique modality in schools of social work with the continued drive toward generalist curricula and emphasis on producing generalist trained practitioners. One result of the lack of focus on method-specific study is the dearth of practitioners adequately trained to facilitate groups in professional settings. Group work writers cite the numbers of field instructors unable to provide adequate supervision for students practicing group work in the field as a result of a lack of group specific education. Fewer practitioners are able to share their expertise in group work with colleagues or assume positions as instructors of group work. Organizations are increasingly pressed to provide services for greater numbers of clients with expedience and in a cost-effective manner. I am reminded of the social work student who came to class one day and announced she needed a purpose for her new group, which was to meet the following week. When probed for details, the student shared her anxiety over facilitating a group of *thirty* members of varying age, race and ethnicity, all with different needs. As she lamented to the class, what purpose could there possibly be for a collection of that many people? Member needs, issues of confidentiality, group composition, and certainly articulation of a group purpose never entered the discussion with agency administration when offering the assignment to the social work intern. Sadly, the student's story is not uncommon in those brought from the front lines and shared by MSW students in my group work classes. The use of groups as an organizational cost-cutting device continues to proliferate in social work. Students of group work continue to be offered field assignments that do not value the skills they are being taught in Master's level group work instruction.

Another story from the field involves a student who co-facilitated a weekly group for parents and their adolescent children in her first year field placement. Her assignment consisted of a scripted curriculum which had been utilized by the agency to great effect, according to her field instructor. Her co-facilitator had neither group work training nor inclination toward mutual aid groups. The social work student, picking up on cues she had learned about in group work class, attempted repeatedly to deviate from her scripted curriculum in response to spontaneous interactions among group members arising from the material presented in the sessions. The student perceived the members' interactions as material for fostering empathy and mutual aid in the group. She was reminded by her co-facilitator that the group did not have time to talk but should get back to the curriculum; perhaps there would be time for group members to continue the discussion after the group session. The student's story prompted a lively discussion in class about the place of mutual aid in curriculum-driven groups. The increase in organizations utilizing curriculum-driven groups, short-term programs, and professionals other than social group workers to facilitate groups implies a lack of understanding for the value of mutual aid, the development of empathy, and the problem-solving process as core concepts in the growth of individuals through the group process.

Given this litany of concerns and the field experiences to back them up, I am troubled by but empathize with students' questions regarding the utility of the concepts, values, and skills of group work as laid out in Kurland and Salmon's text. As a former administrator and practitioner of groups I am all too aware of the various environmental constraints to the high standards for group work promoted by the *Teaching* book. How does one adequately plan a group when not given any opportunity to explore prospective members' needs; when purpose is not considered of value by the host organization; when resources are not made available to accommodate members with special needs; when co-facilitators are brought into the group without any advanced notice to the group members, with little or no pre-group planning, and often little if any group work training; when groups are formed to meet agency numbers rather than client needs . . . the list is endless as any group worker practitioner will attest. I am challenged with how to address their concerns but by not addressing them fully I am only adding to the problem. By burying my head in the text and refusing to see the contemporary constraints to practice I am doing a disservice to both the text and the reality of my students' experiences. I think Kurland and Salmon would agree that the best (and only) way through a problem is to "sit in the mess" of it with the group and explore the many facets of the problem in order to come to some resolution helpful to all concerned. So I sit in the mess of group work with my arts students downtown and my social work students uptown. We discuss the challenges and constraints to group work and we look at examples from practice to inform our dilemma. After all is said and done, I find myself going back to *Teaching a Methods Course*. For as was shared with me by the two gifted social work instructors who wrote the text and as I share with my students, it is only by teaching (and learning) the ideal that we can see what is possible. Once we know what can be gained for the groups we facilitate and why the process of carefully planned, comprehensive group work is so important, we can better understand how to creatively manage the constraints to effective practice. Ultimately, we owe that much to our group members.

If I may be permitted a personal note, it is to offer a heartfelt thank you to Robert Salmon and Roselle Kurland for providing us with *Teaching a Methods Course in Social Work with Groups*. Their text has given us the courage to embrace the "mess" of group work even while teaching the specific skills, concepts, and values that make it the uniquely powerful tool for change that it is. As I continue on my lifelong journey with group work, my trusty teaching guide remains a constant companion. It keeps me on course, challenging me to reflect on the concepts and values of group work as they apply to my own experiences as a practitioner and encouraging me to use my own voice in the teaching of group work. For that I am profoundly grateful.

REFERENCES

Cohen, C. (1998). Review of *Teaching a methods course in social work with groups* in *Social Work with Groups, 21 (3)*, 75-77.

Kurland, R., and Salmon, R. (1998). *Teaching a methods course in social work with groups*. Alexandria, VA: Council on Social Work Education.

Index

AASWG. *See* Association for the
 Advancement of Social Work
 with Groups (AASWG)
Ability to focus, development of,
 boxing in social group work
 providing, 162-163
Academic goals
 for first grade, 126-127
 for fourth grade, 127
 group purpose and, integration of,
 125-126
 for kindergarten, 126
Acceptance, 70-71
Activity(ies), use of, in group work
 practice among campers,
 144-147
Advance group work practice course,
 94-95
Advanced group work practitioners,
 education of
 organizational insight and, 91-104
 challenge facing, 95-96
 introduction to, 91-92
 practice examples, 98-101
 skills for organizational
 intervention in, 101-102
Aid, mutual. *See* Mutual aid
American Association of Group
 Workers, 11
Anderson, J., 76
Anderson, K., 199
Angelou, M., 188
Annual Symposium on Social Work
 with Groups, 93
Appreciation, by group workers, 81-82
Association for the Advancement of
 Social Work with Groups
 (AASWG), xxvi,10,11,29,
 87,93

Annual Symposium of, 18
Fourteenth Annual Symposium of,
 Plenary Presentation of, 2
26th Annual Symposium of, 35
2005 Annual Symposium of, 19
Auerbach, C., 3-4,93

Belief(s), of group workers, 78-81
Bereavement support, group-related,
 for spouses grieving loss of
 partner to cancer, 259-278.
 See also Group bereavement
 support, for spouses grieving
 loss of partner to cancer
Bindler, S.R., 65
Birnbaum, M., 3-4,93
Bitel, M.C., xvii,96,279
Blumenthal, L., 135-136
Bold being, 49-50
Boxing, in social group work, with
 high-risk and offender youth
 ability to focus development,
 162-163
 attributes of, 154-171
 commitment taught by, 163-164
 defense as metaphor in, 159-161
 described, 152-154
 discipline provided by, 158-159
 impulse control improved by,
 161-162
 meaning offered by, 163-164
 mutual aid fostered by, 168-171
 new identity provided by, 154-158
 patience improved by, 161-162
 respect taught by, 165
 safety promoted by, 158
 stress relieved by, 165-168

BOOK ORDER FORM!

Order a copy of this book with this form or online at:
http://www.HaworthPress.com/store/product.asp?sku= 5934

Making Joyful Noise
The Art, Science, and Soul of Group Work

—— in softbound at $30.00 ISBN-13: 978-0-7890-3238-6 / ISBN-10: 0-7890-3238-4.
—— in hardbound at $50.00 ISBN-13: 978-0-7890-3237-9 / ISBN-10: 0-7890-3237-6.

COST OF BOOKS _____

POSTAGE & HANDLING _____
US: $4.00 for first book & $1.50
for each additional book
Outside US: $5.00 for first book
& $2.00 for each additional book.

SUBTOTAL _____

In Canada: add 7% GST. _____

STATE TAX _____
CA, IL, IN, MN, NJ, NY, OH, PA & SD residents
please add appropriate local sales tax.

FINAL TOTAL _____
If paying in Canadian funds, convert
using the current exchange rate,
UNESCO coupons welcome.

❑ BILL ME LATER:
Bill-me option is good on US/Canada/
Mexico orders only; not good to jobbers,
wholesalers, or subscription agencies.

❑ Signature _____

❑ Payment Enclosed: $_____

❑ PLEASE CHARGE TO MY CREDIT CARD:
❑ Visa ❑ MasterCard ❑ AmEx ❑ Discover
❑ Diner's Club ❑ Eurocard ❑ JCB

Account #_____

Exp Date_____

Signature_____
(Prices in US dollars and subject to change without notice.)

PLEASE PRINT ALL INFORMATION OR ATTACH YOUR BUSINESS CARD

Name

Address

City   State/Province   Zip/Postal Code

Country

Tel   Fax

E-Mail

May we use your e-mail address for confirmations and other types of information? ❑ Yes ❑ No We appreciate receiving
your e-mail address. Haworth would like to e-mail special discount offers to you, as a preferred customer.
We will never share, rent, or exchange your e-mail address. We regard such actions as an invasion of your privacy.

Order from your **local bookstore** or directly from
The Haworth Press, Inc. 10 Alice Street, Binghamton, New York 13904-1580 • USA
Call our toll-free number (1-800-429-6784) / Outside US/Canada: (607) 722-5857
Fax: 1-800-895-0582 / Outside US/Canada: (607) 771-0012
E-mail your order to us: orders@HaworthPress.com

For orders outside US and Canada, you may wish to order through your local
sales representative, distributor, or bookseller.
For information, see http://HaworthPress.com/distributors

(Discounts are available for individual orders in US and Canada only, not booksellers/distributors.)

Please photocopy this form for your personal use.
www.HaworthPress.com

BOF06